The FACE Yoga journal

Transform Your Face, Mind & Life in 2 Minutes a Day

Danielle Collins

First published in the UK and USA in 2021 by
Watkins, an imprint of Watkins Media Limited
Unit 11, Shepperton House, 83–93 Shepperton Road
London N1 3DF

enquiries@watkinspublishing.com

Commissioning Editor: Fiona Robertson
Editorial Assistant: Brittany Willis
Head of Design: Glen Wilkins
Commissioned artwork: Glen Wilkins
Production: Uzma Taj
Typeset: JCS Publishing Services Ltd

A CIP record for this book is available from the British Library

ISBN: 978-1-78678-533-6

10 9 8 7 6 5 4 3 2

Printed in Turkey

Publisher's Note: Please work to your own level with all Face Yoga techniques, don't massage over broken or inflamed skin and consult your doctor first if you have any medical or skin conditions.

www.watkinspublishing.com

Contents

About the Author

Danielle Collins is the world leading Face Yoga expert and a renowned Yoga and Wellbeing Coach. She believes in helping and inspiring people to look and feel the best version of themselves using simple, natural and effective techniques.

After being diagnosed with ME in her early 20s and being bedridden, with no formal treatment for the illness, she began to explore natural therapies and she fully recovered in 18 months. This journey led to her founding The Danielle Collins Face Yoga Method, and she now offers international teacher training certifications and has teachers sharing her techniques all over the globe.

Danielle's Face Yoga videos, courses and products are enjoyed by millions of people who love her encouraging and calm manner and her philosophy of beauty, starting from the inside out. Over the last 17 years, Danielle has been featured in hundreds of leading newspapers and magazines and is a regular on TV and radio. She loves building community and sharing her wellness techniques, and this can be seen in the popularity of her YouTube videos and social media platforms. She is the author of *Danielle Collins' Face Yoga* which has been translated into 12 languages.

Danielle is the mum to two lovely little girls, Lucia and Lilia. Danielle and her husband Bruce feel so blessed to be raising them in the beautiful city of Bath in the UK.

Ways to connect with Danielle:

Website (products, courses and teacher training):
    www.faceyogaexpert.com

- @faceyogaexpert
- The Face Yoga Expert
- The Face Yoga Expert
- faceyogaexpert
- @faceyogaexpert
- The Face Yoga Expert
- Danielle Collins

It All Starts Here

You are about to embark on an exciting journey. A journey that will last a whole year and hopefully a lifetime.

I can't promise you it's going to be easy. I can't promise that you will always like the thoughts, feelings and revelations that come to the surface as you start to understand more about your face, mind, body and soul. But this is what I *can* promise you: by this time next year, you will be proud of what you have achieved. You will love that your skin looks healthy and glowing. Most importantly, you will have to hand a toolbox of techniques for a firm, lifted face, a calmer mind and a more balanced body – which you can use for life.

But I can only promise you this if you show up every day. Even the days when you are busy, or when you feel tired, down or fed up, or when you feel like it's not worth the effort and you have zero motivation. All you need to commit to is 2 minutes per day. You can do more, of course (and I would highly recommend that you do), but when you really can't manage any more, 2 minutes is perfect.

Of course, it's inevitable you will miss some days, weeks or months. If this is the case, just pick up exactly where you left off and know that's really okay!

Let's do this together. This year, you have me by your side every single day.

My "why"

So why have I written this journal?

Well, let's start with the big "why". This is my reason for all I do. When I was 21, I suffered from the chronic illness ME, which left me bedridden and housebound for the large part of 18 months. It was equally the worst and best time of my life. It was lonely, dark and painful. But it was also transformative. I not only transformed from a stressed-out and chronically ill patient to a fully recovered and healed human, but I also gained a deep purpose to help others. During those long days of pain, I remember clearly saying to myself that when I recover from this, I will make it my life's work to help others heal. I didn't know exactly how I would do it but I knew that was all I wanted. Even to this day, the reason I teach, write and share daily is because I know there are so many people who want to feel healthier and happier. Helping, healing and teaching is my soul purpose – or, as it's so beautifully called in yoga, my *dharma*.

Okay, now let's delve in to the "why" of *The Face Yoga Journal*. I was lying in the bath one day thinking how wonderful Face Yoga and simple daily wellness rituals are, yet we often don't stick to them or do them enough. As I thought about the reasons for this, which I have heard from my clients in my clinics, classes, presentations and teacher trainings, as well as from the millions of people who enjoy The Danielle Collins' Face Yoga Method online, I managed to compile (once I was out the bath!) seven key reasons.

1. **Lack of time.** This is the main reason that people give for not doing daily Face Yoga or self-care. We live in a fast-paced world where it is so easy to put everything and everyone else first. This journal is designed to help you even if time is short. All you need to dedicate to yourself is 2 minutes minimum a day. Each week you are given a new Face Yoga move that takes 1 minute, and then you can spend your second minute on a wellness technique, such as setting an intention or your gratitude practice. Ideally, you spend a few more minutes (probably around 5) on a Monday and Sunday filling in your weekly activities. My hope is you will notice how amazing you look and feel by taking just 2 minutes each day, and quickly you will realize that spending around 30 minutes a day on Face Yoga and wellness will really help you to feel your best.

2. **Lack of motivation.** This journal is designed to help you with exactly that – it uses many tools and activities to spark motivation. One of the best ways to do this, though, is simply to begin! There is no better motivation than feeling great and looking great, and this will start to happen within the first few weeks of your Face Yoga practice.

3. **Disbelief of results.** Take before and after pictures every week. This helps quantify your results so well.

4. **Impatience.** This is a journey, not a quick fix. Great results do happen but it takes daily practice and dedication.

5. **Not worrying about looking older.** This is great! But I would still recommend you do Face Yoga to feel good.

6. **Worrying too much about looking older.** Sometimes we can get ourselves so anxious that it paralyzes us and we take no action, or the opposite is true and we take too much action and become obsessed. This journal will guide you to become balanced in your practice.

7. **Lack of accountability.** Each day write down when you did your Face Yoga and for how long, as this means you will hold yourself accountable. If it helps, visualize that I am with you, supporting you and checking your daily progress!

How to use *The Face Yoga Journal*

The Seasons

This journal is divided into four seasons. These seasons aren't intended to match the traditional seasons as we know them; depending on where you live in the world and at what point of the year you start this journal, the season will vary. They are instead intended to neatly separate your year into four themes to provide a nice start and pause point every 13 weeks. Your goal is to complete 52 weeks. So even if you start this mid-way through your calendar year and even if you miss a few weeks here and there, that's okay. Simply pick up where you left off and never feel guilty!

Your four seasons are:

Season 1: Love your face

Season 2: Energize your face

Season 3: Lift your face

Season 4: Soothe your face

For each season, at the start of each of the 13 weeks, I will give you five things that relate to that season:

1. Your happiness chemical

Each season is connected to a happiness chemical in the brain. All the techniques are aimed to help boost and, where appropriate, balance this chemical. This is, of course, done in a very subtle and simplified way, as these brain chemicals are quite complex. But here is a little more information for you:

Season 1: Love your face: Oxytocin

Oxytocin is known as the love chemical. We release this when we are cuddling, giving kind words to ourselves and others, kissing, making love, holding hands and stroking pets.

Season 2: Energize your face: Endorphins

Endorphins are known as the feel-good chemicals. We release these when exercising, laughing, doing fun activities and using essential oils.

Season 3: Lift your face: Dopamine

Dopamine is known as the reward chemical. We release it when doing a wellness activity, making love, eating pleasurable food or ticking off a to-do list.

Season 4: Soothe your face: Serotonin

Serotonin is known as the mood-stabilizing chemical. We release it when exercising, meditating, being in the present moment and being around nature.

2. The chakras

The word *chakra* means "wheel" in Sanskrit (origin: India). Chakras are believed to be spinning vortexes or discs of energy that, when open, aligned or balanced, means we are in good physical, mental and emotional health.

There are seven main chakras that correspond to different points of the spinal column and in each of the four seasons you will learn a little more about how to balance one or two of them through your Face Yoga and wellness rituals.

Season 1: Love your face: heart chakra and solar plexus chakra

Heart chakra: located in the centre of our chest area. This chakra is connected to our beauty, love and compassion for ourselves and others.
Solar plexus chakra: located just above the navel and below the rib cage. This chakra is linked to our power, self-worth, intuition, soul purpose and self-esteem.

Season 2: Energize your face: crown chakra and sacral chakra

Crown chakra: located at the top of the head. This chakra is connected to our higher consciousness (to take us beyond our personal preoccupations) and is about our connection with the universe as a whole.
Sacral chakra: located in the lower abdominal area, 7.5cm/3in below the navel. This chakra is connected to our sexuality, creativity and emotion.

Season 3: Lift your face: third eye chakra

Third eye chakra: located between the eyebrows. This chakra is linked to our intuition, wisdom, awareness and spiritual insight.

Season 4: Soothe your face: root chakra and throat chakra
Root chakra: located at the base of the spine. This chakra is related to how grounded, safe and secure we feel and is linked to a sense of being rather than doing.
Throat chakra: located in the lower neck area. This chakra is about our expression, communication and speaking our truth from our inner authentic voice.

3. Colours
Each of the chakras has a corresponding colour, and the colours follow the order of the rainbow:

Root: red
Sacral: orange
Solar plexus: yellow
Heart: green
Throat: blue
Third eye: indigo
Crown: white (sometimes a pale purple)

Throughout your year, each season will focus on one or two colours, which also match the chakras of that season.

Season 1: green and yellow
Season 2: white (or pale purple) and orange
Season 3: indigo
Season 4: red and blue

By incorporating these colours into your life, you are helping to balance your chakras and enhance wellness. Some ways you can use this colour therapy:

- Wear the colour as clothes or jewellery.
- Surround yourself with these colours in your home – such as the decor, accessories and flowers.
- Meditate with these colours. Simply see these colours in your mind, focus on an item or crystal with this colour or tune in to the chakra which corresponds to this colour.

4. Crystals

Crystals are, put simply, a solid formation made of atoms which have an orderly and repeated arrangement.

Although there is still little scientific evidence to prove the healing, spiritual and wellness benefits of crystals, they have been used traditionally for many thousands of years for positively interacting with chakras due their unique vibrational qualities. If nothing else, they are calming to be around, wonderful to touch and beautiful to look at. And let's face it, all those things boost our wellbeing!

Each season I have recommended a few crystals which link nicely to the themes, chakras, colours and Face Yoga techniques of that season. This doesn't mean you have to run out and buy each one, but if you happen to have any of these, bring them into your personal space or somewhere you will see them regularly for the 13 weeks of that season. A note here: please ensure your crystals are ethically sourced, that you cleanse them regularly and use ones that you are intuitively attracted to. If you do have them already or you choose to purchase them, here are four things you may like to do with them:

1. Place the crystals on a shelf in your house (they can be particularly nice in the bedroom or by the bath) so they are in your mental, physical and spiritual space.
2. Hold the crystals in your hand while you meditate or breathe, or place them in front of you whilst doing your Face Yoga techniques.
3. Wear them as jewellery – as rings, necklaces or bracelets – or even place one in your pocket.
4. Use them as a roller or gua sha tool (never use crystals on the face that are not for use on the face and look for good-quality rollers and gua shas – you can find these in my online shop). Crystals such as jade, rose quartz and clear quartz are wonderful for the skin.

Here are my recommended crystals. Please note: there are many crystals for each chakra and I have just chosen one for each because I resonate with these particular stones. If you prefer others, or would like your crystal colour to match the colour of the chakra, please use what suits you.

Season 1: Love your face
Rose quartz for the heart chakra
Yellow topaz for the solar plexus chakra

Season 2: Energize your face
Clear quartz for the crown chakra
Sunstone for the sacral chakra

Season 3: Lift your face
Amethyst for the third eye chakra

Season 4: Soothe your face
Black tourmaline for the root chakra
Turquoise for the throat chakra

5. Mantras

A mantra is a phrase you repeat frequently to have a positive impact on your mindset, your physical body and, of course, your face. Each season, the mantra chosen is designed to reflect the seasonal theme and chakra. I recommend you say these in your mind or out loud *at least* once a day for each of the 13 weeks, and more if you can. I recommend saying it just before you get out of bed, as what we say to ourselves in those first few seconds has a huge impact on our wellness for the rest of the day. Other great times to repeat these are whilst doing your Face Yoga, whilst taking a deep breath, whilst holding or wearing your crystal or whenever you feel in need of a boost mentally, emotionally or physically.

Season 1: Love your face: "Love is all around me, within me and radiating from me."

Season 2: Energize your face: "I know and understand that I deserve to feel great."

Season 3: Lift your face: "I see, trust and know my own inner and outer beauty."

Season 4: Soothe your face: "I speak words that resonate with who I truly am."

The Weeks

Weekly theme

Over the 52 weeks, you have 52 themes – one per week. The themes will guide everything from the Face Yoga moves you will do to the wellness hacks and everything in between. Each week I will explain exactly why the chosen theme is important and how to use it.

Weekly Face Yoga

Now let's address Face Yoga itself because it is a large and important part of this journal. This is a very brief mention as more will be shared with you weekly throughout the year.

Each week you will be introduced to a new Face Yoga technique which focuses on one part of the face and is linked to your seasonal and weekly theme.

Face Yoga

The Danielle Collins Face Yoga Method, which is what you will be doing daily in this journal, is a natural way of looking and feeling healthy, glowing and youthful. It is safe, non-invasive and rooted in traditional Indian and Chinese healing techniques with modern, science-based research. I have taught this technique to millions of people around the world including celebrities, and on many major TV shows. When I created this method over 16 years ago my goal was (and still is) to help you have a simple and easy yet effective tool in your own hands that you can use daily.

Face Yoga combines facial exercises, facial massage, acupressure, facial relaxation and, of course, wellbeing. Face Yoga lifts and firms the face, helps smooth lines, relaxes tension and helps you to look the best version of you.

To get good results, you need to keep it up daily. You also need a mirror, clean hands, a clean face and a little serum (such as Fusion by Danielle Collins) prior to starting. Breathe deeply throughout. It's key to wear SPF every day when outside, whatever the weather – this is the best thing you can do for your skin!

You can use the 52 Face Yoga techniques in the journal in three ways:

1. Do 1 minute per day: Do the weekly 1-minute Face Yoga technique daily.
2. Do 1–52 minutes: This is about accumulation, so each week you will be adding 1 more minute to your routine until week 52 when you will have a 52-minute routine. After you complete the year you can then decide how long suits you. Usually, a realistic time whilst getting the best results is between 10 and 30 minutes daily.
3. Do 1 minute plus your usual routine: Do your usual daily Face Yoga routine plus the 1-minute daily technique suggested each week. Use the space in this journal to record what Face Yoga you do and when.

Please note: if you have any of my other books, courses, apps or DVDs, you can use the techniques in this journal as well as or instead of the techniques you have already. Variety can boost our motivation and is great for our muscles, so it's up to you – they are all equally good!

Weekly wellness hack

This is a quick and simple tip or action that complements your Face Yoga. Feeling good on the inside can help you to look great on the outside. Please try to do your wellness hack every week; it really will help you get the best results. Some hacks aren't by any means groundbreaking and many you may already do or have heard of before, but they are achievable and get good results. They may, in some cases, be life-changing and deeply transformative, so stay open-minded. Some of these hacks you may do just for one day, one week or all year. And some that resonate with you at a soul level will become part of your routine for life.

Weekly positive statement

Every week you will see an uplifting statement in your journal. There is no action for you to take on this, so use it as you choose. Simply take 3–5 seconds to read it once, read it multiple times during the day or week, think about it and how you can apply it to your daily life or write it down and stick it somewhere in your home where you will see it often. As with many aspects of this journal, see what resonates with you and be intuitive daily on what your mental, physical, emotional, spiritual and aesthetic needs are.

My positive word for the week

The next three sections explain a little action that is required from you each week. Choosing a positive word can set the tone for the week. So how do you choose one? My favourite way is to close my eyes, take a deep breath and simply ask myself: "Which word do I need in my life this week?" Listen to your gut-instinct answer and go with that, even if on the surface there seems no initial reason for it. If you're struggling, browse over the theme, wellness hacks, positive statement and Face Yoga technique for the week and use that to inspire your word.

The way I want to feel this week

Once again, simplicity and intuition are key here. Taking a deep breath (in through the nose for 4 and out through the nose for 6), ask yourself: "How do I want to feel this week?" Listen to your first answer. You may find you use the same answer for many weeks or even for the whole year, and that's fine if that is what your intuition is telling you each week.

My reason for doing Face Yoga this week

The answer to this question may vary every week or it might be the same for an entire season. One of the best ways to keep motivated is to really and honestly know *why* you are doing Face Yoga. The word honestly is key here. If you do it to reduce a deep wrinkle on your face, then write that. If you do it because you want to balance out your work stress, jot it down. It doesn't matter the reason, but it does matter that it's truthful and from the heart.

What went well this week

This is your chance to celebrate anything that went well about your Face Yoga and wellness routine!

What didn't go so well this week

In many ways I see this as one of the most powerful exercises. Acknowledgement of and sitting with any negative feelings, even for a few seconds, allows them to pass through us rather than simply get stuck. It also teaches us the art of getting comfortable with discomfort. What you write may be focused on Face Yoga but equally may be about an emotion, a lack of emotion, a difficult person or a stressful event. Whatever it is, write it down and feel it, even if this isn't nice to do. Then take a deep breath in and out through your nose and let it move through your mind and body, maybe even let it go, depending on whether you're ready to. Know that true wellbeing doesn't mean being motivated and happy all the time; it comes from acknowledging difficult feelings, hard times and perceived failures, and understanding that "this too shall pass".

The Days

Today's intention
Your daily Face Yoga and wellness goals should be intentional. When we know where we want to go, we are more likely to get there.

When I did my Face Yoga today
This is an easy tick box to keep you accountable and motivated; it helps you to celebrate your dedication. Simply tick what time of day you did your Face Yoga technique(s).

The areas I worked on today
Each day, note down which areas of the face you focused on. If you are just doing the 1-minute technique daily, then the answer will be the same all week. But if you use other techniques, you will be ticking multiple or all boxes.

What I am most grateful for today
I deeply believe that one of the best things we can do for our mind, body and face is to be thankful. Thankful for where we have been, where we are and where we are going in our journey of life. It brings happiness, blessings, positivity and results. Each day, choose one thing, moment, person or practice in your life that you are grateful for. The art of writing this down is so powerful.

Season 1
Love your face

Happiness chemical: oxytocin
Chakras: heart chakra and solar plexus chakra
Crystals: rose quartz and yellow topaz
Colours: green and yellow

Mantra: "Love is all around me, within me and radiating from me."

There is one thing that I want you to always feel but still focus on over the next 13 weeks, and that is love. Love for your face, love for your yourself, love for your mind, love for your body and love for the people and things around you. This really is at the root of Danielle Collins' Face Yoga Method and everything I stand for. I honestly believe that when we are in a state of unconditional love, we are happier, healthier and we glow inside and out.

Your goal over the next three months is to increase your understanding, respect and adoration for yourself. This may be uncomfortable or difficult at times but that is part of the journey. Just sit with the discomfort and let it move through you when it's ready. According to neuroscience, our brain is hardwired to remember the negative events more than the positive; we are not designed to always be happy in order to protect us against danger and, in essence, to help humanity survive. So if you aren't brimming with self-love all the time, that's normal. But it is important to remember that part of surviving and, even more than that, part of thriving, is to have a toolbox of techniques to help us feel love and happiness much of the time too.

The wellness hacks, the Face Yoga techniques and your gratitude practice will all help you with this. Every time you touch your face this season, feel the love running through your hands and radiating on to your face. I promise that when you move from criticism to love through physical touch and positive words, your face will look healthier and more youthful.

Focusing on the heart chakra, which can be done by surrounding yourself with the colour green and using a rose quartz crystal, helps you connect to your beauty, love and compassion for yourself and others. The solar plexus chakra is linked to our power, self-worth, intuition, soul purpose and self-esteem. Using a yellow topaz and the colour yellow can help activate this chakra.

All your weekly themes are focused on loving your face. Each one has been specifically designed to help promote self-love and compassion.

Week 1. Understanding

This week your focus is on getting to know your face, your facial habits and your breath. We often hold stress and tension in certain areas of the face, being aware of some parts and disconnected to others. We can also spend a lot of time criticizing our face. This week, do the Face Yoga technique at least once a day to have a true understanding of your face, to feel the wonderful benefits of deep breathing and inner reflection and, above all, to feel grateful for your face. You may like to hold your rose quartz crystal in your hand for the first part of the Face Yoga move.

TECHNIQUE OF THE WEEK
The Face Understanding Technique

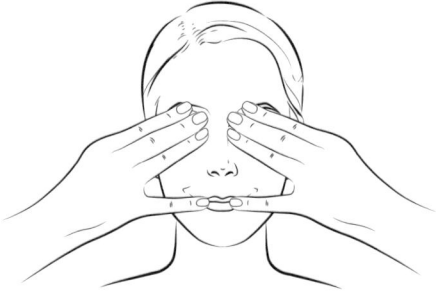

1. Close your eyes and take a deep breath. Using your mind, focus on each part of your face for 15 seconds, starting at the forehead. Simply notice what each part feels like, without judgement.

2. Do the same thing again but consciously relaxing tension and stress from each area for 15 seconds.

3. With a relaxed face, gently place three fingers of both hands over your eyes. Place your little fingers on your closed lips and your thumbs lightly in your ears so that three senses are closed off and you can breathe only through the nose (avoid if nasal breathing doesn't work for you). Do this for 30 seconds, or longer if you choose.

Benefits: The first part of this technique is one of the most important practices you can do for your face to prevent and soften lines, wrinkles and discomfort. The second part gives you a chance to use one of the most powerful wellness tools you have – your breath – with an added benefit of inward reflection and peace as you close off some senses.

> **Weekly wellness hack** Every time you pass a mirror, stop and do two things. Firstly, scan your face visually without judgement, noticing where you are holding tension or creasing your face, then consciously relax this part. Secondly, say to yourself three times "I am enough". This is so simple but it can prevent and reduce stress lines as well as boost self-love.

My Positive Word for the Week:

....

The Way I Want to Feel this Week:

....

My Reason for Doing Face Yoga this Week:

....

"Please remember it's a privilege to grow older. Not everyone has this privilege."

MONDAY

Today's intention:

....

When I did my Face Yoga today:

AM practice .... minutes   PM practice .... minutes

The areas I worked on today:

☐ Forehead   ☐ Eyes   ☐ Cheeks   ☐ Mouth   ☐ Jaw   ☐ Neck   ☐ Wellness

What I am most grateful for today:

....

....

TUESDAY

Today's intention:

....

When I did my Face Yoga today:

AM practice .... minutes   PM practice .... minutes

The areas I worked on today:

☐ Forehead   ☐ Eyes   ☐ Cheeks   ☐ Mouth   ☐ Jaw   ☐ Neck   ☐ Wellness

What I am most grateful for today:

....

....

WEDNESDAY

Today's intention:

....

When I did my Face Yoga today:

AM practice .... minutes   PM practice .... minutes

The areas I worked on today:

☐ Forehead ☐ Eyes ☐ Cheeks ☐ Mouth ☐ Jaw ☐ Neck ☐ Wellness

What I am most grateful for today:

....

....

THURSDAY

Today's intention:

....

When I did my Face Yoga today:

AM practice .... minutes   PM practice .... minutes

The areas I worked on today:

☐ Forehead ☐ Eyes ☐ Cheeks ☐ Mouth ☐ Jaw ☐ Neck ☐ Wellness

What I am most grateful for today:

....

....

FRIDAY

Today's intention:

....

When I did my Face Yoga today:

AM practice .... minutes   PM practice .... minutes

The areas I worked on today:

☐ Forehead   ☐ Eyes   ☐ Cheeks   ☐ Mouth   ☐ Jaw   ☐ Neck   ☐ Wellness

What I am most grateful for today:

....

....

SATURDAY

Today's intention:

....

When I did my Face Yoga today:

AM practice .... minutes   PM practice .... minutes

The areas I worked on today:

☐ Forehead   ☐ Eyes   ☐ Cheeks   ☐ Mouth   ☐ Jaw   ☐ Neck   ☐ Wellness

What I am most grateful for today:

....

....

SUNDAY

Today's intention:

....

When I did my Face Yoga today:

AM practice .... minutes   PM practice .... minutes

The areas I worked on today:

☐ Forehead   ☐ Eyes   ☐ Cheeks   ☐ Mouth   ☐ Jaw   ☐ Neck   ☐ Wellness

What I am most grateful for today:

....

....

What Went Well this Week:

....

....

What Didn't Go so Well this Week:

....

....

Week 2. Motivation

This week it's all about setting intentions and feeling motivated for the rest of the year. Each day this week while doing your Face Yoga, be clear in your mind *why* you are embarking on your Face Yoga journey. This week's Face Yoga evokes instant feelings of calm and softens lines, both of which are highly motivating – because when you feel and look good, and you love your face, you want to do more.

TECHNIQUE OF THE WEEK
The Forehead Motivating Technique

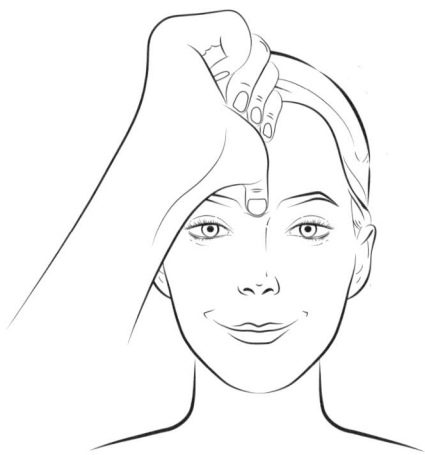

1. Place the pad of your thumb in the space between your eyebrows yet slightly below, just on the bridge of your nose. Gently smooth your thumb upward about 3–5 centimetres, then flick it off.

2. Go back to the starting position and continue for 1 minute.

Benefits: This helps to relax tension in the procerus muscle between your eyebrows which helps prevent glabellar lines (or number 11 lines) which are formed from stress-related expressions. It also helps to boost blood flow to the area for brighter skin, as well as stimulating a calming acupressure point.

> **Weekly wellness hack** Holding on to clutter and living in a messy environment negatively affects our mental health and leaves us demotivated. Each day this week, dedicate a little time to clear out unwanted or unnecessary things that don't bring you joy or are of no use and tidy up as many areas of your home as you can.

My Positive Word for the Week:

....

The Way I Want to Feel this Week:

....

My Reason for Doing Face Yoga this Week:

....

"It's your life. You choose how to live. Remember that."

MONDAY

Today's intention:

....

When I did my Face Yoga today:

AM practice .... minutes   PM practice .... minutes

The areas I worked on today:

☐ Forehead   ☐ Eyes   ☐ Cheeks   ☐ Mouth   ☐ Jaw   ☐ Neck   ☐ Wellness

What I am most grateful for today:

....

....

TUESDAY

Today's intention:

....

When I did my Face Yoga today:

AM practice .... minutes   PM practice .... minutes

The areas I worked on today:

☐ Forehead   ☐ Eyes   ☐ Cheeks   ☐ Mouth   ☐ Jaw   ☐ Neck   ☐ Wellness

What I am most grateful for today:

....

....

WEDNESDAY

Today's intention:

....

When I did my Face Yoga today:

AM practice .... minutes   PM practice .... minutes

The areas I worked on today:

☐ Forehead ☐ Eyes ☐ Cheeks ☐ Mouth ☐ Jaw ☐ Neck ☐ Wellness

What I am most grateful for today:

....

....

THURSDAY

Today's intention:

....

When I did my Face Yoga today:

AM practice .... minutes   PM practice .... minutes

The areas I worked on today:

☐ Forehead ☐ Eyes ☐ Cheeks ☐ Mouth ☐ Jaw ☐ Neck ☐ Wellness

What I am most grateful for today:

....

....

FRIDAY

Today's intention:

....

When I did my Face Yoga today:

AM practice .... minutes   PM practice .... minutes

The areas I worked on today:

☐ Forehead   ☐ Eyes   ☐ Cheeks   ☐ Mouth   ☐ Jaw   ☐ Neck   ☐ Wellness

What I am most grateful for today:

....

....

SATURDAY

Today's intention:

....

When I did my Face Yoga today:

AM practice .... minutes   PM practice .... minutes

The areas I worked on today:

☐ Forehead   ☐ Eyes   ☐ Cheeks   ☐ Mouth   ☐ Jaw   ☐ Neck   ☐ Wellness

What I am most grateful for today:

....

....

SUNDAY

Today's intention:

....

When I did my Face Yoga today:

AM practice .... minutes   PM practice .... minutes

The areas I worked on today:

☐ Forehead ☐ Eyes ☐ Cheeks ☐ Mouth ☐ Jaw ☐ Neck ☐ Wellness

What I am most grateful for today:

....

....

What Went Well this Week:

....

....

What Didn't Go so Well this Week:

....

....

Week 3. Awakening

This week your focus is on awakening your skin, your gratitude and your mind. Your Face Yoga technique is focused on the eye area and when you wake up this area, this helps the rest of your face and mind feel awakened too. You are now in week three so hopefully you are feeling more awakened to the power of wellness, thankfulness and skincare and are feeling a shift in all these areas. Try wearing yellow this week to awaken your solar plexus chakra, which can give you energy and help your intuition.

TECHNIQUE OF THE WEEK
The Eye Awakening Technique

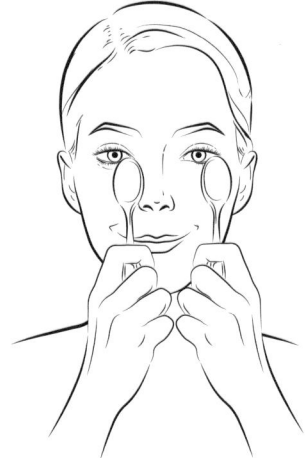

1. Keep two teaspoons in the refrigerator. Hold a spoon in each hand and using the curved backs of the spoons, gently press under your eyes for 30 seconds, especially where there is puffiness or dark circles.

2. Apply a small drop of serum or eye cream around your eyes. Gently smooth the spoons above your eyebrows (starting at the inner edge of your eyebrows) then around your eyes, under your eyes and back to the starting position. Do this for 30 seconds.

Benefits: This massage helps encourage lymphatic drainage and better circulation to reduce and prevent puffiness and dark circles under your eyes. The coolness of the spoons helps to further take down inflammation.

> **Weekly wellness hack** When you wake up and before you even get out of bed each morning this week, simply repeat the words "Thank you" three times. What happens in your mind in the very first few seconds of waking sets the tone for the day.

My Positive Word for the Week:

....

The Way I Want to Feel this Week:

....

My Reason for Doing Face Yoga this Week:

....

"You deserve to be happy."

MONDAY

Today's intention:

....

When I did my Face Yoga today:

AM practice .... minutes   PM practice .... minutes

The areas I worked on today:

☐ Forehead ☐ Eyes ☐ Cheeks ☐ Mouth ☐ Jaw ☐ Neck ☐ Wellness

What I am most grateful for today:

....

....

TUESDAY

Today's intention:

....

When I did my Face Yoga today:

AM practice .... minutes   PM practice .... minutes

The areas I worked on today:

☐ Forehead ☐ Eyes ☐ Cheeks ☐ Mouth ☐ Jaw ☐ Neck ☐ Wellness

What I am most grateful for today:

....

....

WEDNESDAY

Today's intention:

....

When I did my Face Yoga today:

AM practice .... minutes   PM practice .... minutes

The areas I worked on today:

☐ Forehead ☐ Eyes ☐ Cheeks ☐ Mouth ☐ Jaw ☐ Neck ☐ Wellness

What I am most grateful for today:

....

....

THURSDAY

Today's intention:

....

When I did my Face Yoga today:

AM practice .... minutes   PM practice .... minutes

The areas I worked on today:

☐ Forehead ☐ Eyes ☐ Cheeks ☐ Mouth ☐ Jaw ☐ Neck ☐ Wellness

What I am most grateful for today:

....

....

FRIDAY

Today's intention:

....

When I did my Face Yoga today:

AM practice .... minutes   PM practice .... minutes

The areas I worked on today:

☐ Forehead   ☐ Eyes   ☐ Cheeks   ☐ Mouth   ☐ Jaw   ☐ Neck   ☐ Wellness

What I am most grateful for today:

....

....

SATURDAY

Today's intention:

....

When I did my Face Yoga today:

AM practice .... minutes   PM practice .... minutes

The areas I worked on today:

☐ Forehead   ☐ Eyes   ☐ Cheeks   ☐ Mouth   ☐ Jaw   ☐ Neck   ☐ Wellness

What I am most grateful for today:

....

....

SUNDAY

Today's intention:

....

When I did my Face Yoga today:

AM practice .... minutes   PM practice .... minutes

The areas I worked on today:

☐ Forehead ☐ Eyes ☐ Cheeks ☐ Mouth ☐ Jaw ☐ Neck ☐ Wellness

What I am most grateful for today:

....

....

What Went Well this Week:

....

....

What Didn't Go so Well this Week:

....

....

Week 4. Respect

One of the most positive things you can do for yourself is give yourself respect. True respect involves knowing how special you are, as well as seeing special qualities in others. As you do this week's Face Yoga, have respect for your skin, your muscles, your bones and your blood. This respectful energy helps the face to look and feel happier and healthier. This week really focus on your mantra of the season too to further boost self-respect and self-love: "Love is all around me, within me and radiating from me."

TECHNIQUE OF THE WEEK
The Cheek Respecting Technique

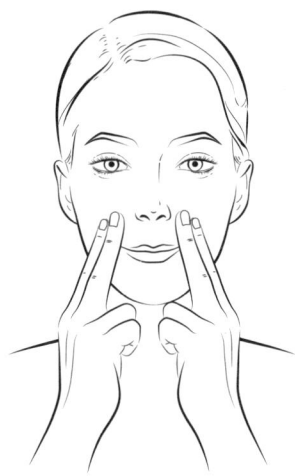

1. With your index and middle fingers starting at your nostrils, moving your hands away from each other, sweep your fingers under the cheek bone then up to your temples. When they reach your temples, lift your fingers off and go back to the starting position.

2. Continue the massage for 1 minute.

Benefits: This is excellent for brightening dull cheeks, easing stress from muscles and lifting the skin. It works by increasing the fresh blood, nutrients and oxygen to the top layer of skin, the epidermis.

> **Weekly wellness hack** During the week, each time you feel uncomfortable, unhappy or unwell, don't ignore it, numb it or try to instantly make yourself feel positive. Take a few minutes to sit with the discomfort and respect why it is there, and then let it pass and dissipate, giving space for positivity to come naturally.

My Positive Word for the Week:

....

The Way I Want to Feel this Week:

....

My Reason for Doing Face Yoga this Week:

....

"Be respectful to yourself and others. We are all healing from things we may not speak about."

MONDAY

Today's intention:

....

When I did my Face Yoga today:

AM practice .... minutes   PM practice .... minutes

The areas I worked on today:

☐ Forehead   ☐ Eyes   ☐ Cheeks   ☐ Mouth   ☐ Jaw   ☐ Neck   ☐ Wellness

What I am most grateful for today:

....

....

TUESDAY

Today's intention:

....

When I did my Face Yoga today:

AM practice .... minutes   PM practice .... minutes

The areas I worked on today:

☐ Forehead   ☐ Eyes   ☐ Cheeks   ☐ Mouth   ☐ Jaw   ☐ Neck   ☐ Wellness

What I am most grateful for today:

....

....

WEDNESDAY

Today's intention:

....

When I did my Face Yoga today:

AM practice .... minutes   PM practice .... minutes

The areas I worked on today:

☐ Forehead ☐ Eyes ☐ Cheeks ☐ Mouth ☐ Jaw ☐ Neck ☐ Wellness

What I am most grateful for today:

....

....

THURSDAY

Today's intention:

....

When I did my Face Yoga today:

AM practice .... minutes   PM practice .... minutes

The areas I worked on today:

☐ Forehead ☐ Eyes ☐ Cheeks ☐ Mouth ☐ Jaw ☐ Neck ☐ Wellness

What I am most grateful for today:

....

....

FRIDAY

Today's intention:

....

When I did my Face Yoga today:

AM practice .... minutes   PM practice .... minutes

The areas I worked on today:

☐ Forehead   ☐ Eyes   ☐ Cheeks   ☐ Mouth   ☐ Jaw   ☐ Neck   ☐ Wellness

What I am most grateful for today:

....

....

SATURDAY

Today's intention:

....

When I did my Face Yoga today:

AM practice .... minutes   PM practice .... minutes

The areas I worked on today:

☐ Forehead   ☐ Eyes   ☐ Cheeks   ☐ Mouth   ☐ Jaw   ☐ Neck   ☐ Wellness

What I am most grateful for today:

....

....

SUNDAY

Today's intention:

....

When I did my Face Yoga today:

AM practice .... minutes   PM practice .... minutes

The areas I worked on today:

☐ Forehead ☐ Eyes ☐ Cheeks ☐ Mouth ☐ Jaw ☐ Neck ☐ Wellness

What I am most grateful for today:

....

....

What Went Well this Week:

....

....

What Didn't Go so Well this Week:

....

....

Week 5. Restoring

This week is all about restoring the face, body and mind. Your Face Yoga technique is great for restoring muscle tone in the lower face, your wellness hack helps you to restore length and strength in your body and as you write your intentions and what you're grateful for this week, aim to focus on ways you can restore your mind.

TECHNIQUE OF THE WEEK
The Mouth Restoring Technique

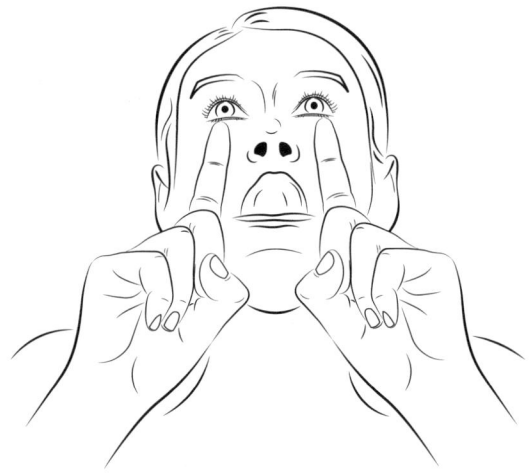

1. Bring the tip of your tongue toward your nose and rest it just above your lips. Then lift the corners of your lips upward slightly. Use your index fingers to smooth any smile lines that have been created around your mouth (plus this will provide a little resistance too). Gently tilt your head back a little if this is comfortable for your neck. Hold for 5 seconds, then lower your head back down.

2. Keep this movement going for 1 minute, holding for 5 seconds at the top each time.

Benefits: This strengthens and restores muscle tone in your cheeks, around your mouth, in the jaw and under the chin. As these muscles build in strength and tone, the skin attached will become smoother, firmer and more lifted.

> **Weekly wellness hack** A few times during the day this week, take note of your posture to restore good alignment. Improved posture reduces back and neck pain, lower face lines and bloating. Good posture aids digestion, helps reduce stress and prevents pain. Relax the shoulders, pull up through the crown of your head and ensure your weight is evenly distributed between both feet.

My Positive Word for the Week:

....

The Way I Want to Feel this Week:

....

My Reason for Doing Face Yoga this Week:

....

"Our greatest wealth is our mental and physical health."

MONDAY

Today's intention:

....

When I did my Face Yoga today:

AM practice .... minutes   PM practice .... minutes

The areas I worked on today:

☐ Forehead   ☐ Eyes   ☐ Cheeks   ☐ Mouth   ☐ Jaw   ☐ Neck   ☐ Wellness

What I am most grateful for today:

....

....

TUESDAY

Today's intention:

....

When I did my Face Yoga today:

AM practice .... minutes   PM practice .... minutes

The areas I worked on today:

☐ Forehead   ☐ Eyes   ☐ Cheeks   ☐ Mouth   ☐ Jaw   ☐ Neck   ☐ Wellness

What I am most grateful for today:

....

....

WEDNESDAY

Today's intention:

....

When I did my Face Yoga today:

AM practice .... minutes   PM practice .... minutes

The areas I worked on today:

☐ Forehead ☐ Eyes ☐ Cheeks ☐ Mouth ☐ Jaw ☐ Neck ☐ Wellness

What I am most grateful for today:

....

....

THURSDAY

Today's intention:

....

When I did my Face Yoga today:

AM practice .... minutes   PM practice .... minutes

The areas I worked on today:

☐ Forehead ☐ Eyes ☐ Cheeks ☐ Mouth ☐ Jaw ☐ Neck ☐ Wellness

What I am most grateful for today:

....

....

FRIDAY

Today's intention:

....

When I did my Face Yoga today:

AM practice .... minutes   PM practice .... minutes

The areas I worked on today:

☐ Forehead   ☐ Eyes   ☐ Cheeks   ☐ Mouth   ☐ Jaw   ☐ Neck   ☐ Wellness

What I am most grateful for today:

....

....

SATURDAY

Today's intention:

....

When I did my Face Yoga today:

AM practice .... minutes   PM practice .... minutes

The areas I worked on today:

☐ Forehead   ☐ Eyes   ☐ Cheeks   ☐ Mouth   ☐ Jaw   ☐ Neck   ☐ Wellness

What I am most grateful for today:

....

....

SUNDAY

Today's intention:

....

When I did my Face Yoga today:

AM practice .... minutes   PM practice .... minutes

The areas I worked on today:

☐ Forehead ☐ Eyes ☐ Cheeks ☐ Mouth ☐ Jaw ☐ Neck ☐ Wellness

What I am most grateful for today:

....

....

What Went Well this Week:

....

....

What Didn't Go so Well this Week:

....

....

Week 6. Support

Feeling supported comes from within but support is also something we need to give to, and receive from, others. This week your Face Yoga technique is wonderful for supporting the muscles in the jaw by releasing any stress they may be holding. Your wellness hack allows you to gain support and give support to others. Take a moment to read this week's quote any time you need a reminder that there is always support if and when you need it.

TECHNIQUE OF THE WEEK
The Jaw Supporting Technique

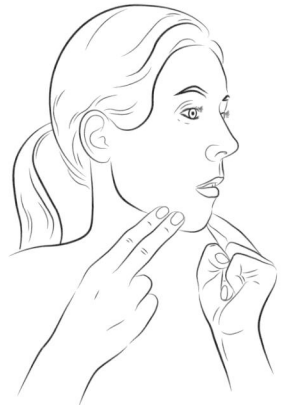

1. Place your index and middle fingers on your chin, under the lip area. Start to massage up the jawline in small circular motions (about 3 circles per spot, then move on) with your hands moving away from each other. Do this for 30 seconds.

2. Place your index fingers in the indentations at the top of the jawbone, under your ear lobes. Press there for 15 seconds.

3. Massage in a circular motion clockwise for 5–10 seconds and then anticlockwise for 5–10 seconds.

Benefits: This is an excellent way to release very common tension and stress from the jaw area. As you relax the tension you are less likely to hold unhelpful expressions which cause lines. You are also boosting circulation and improving muscle tone through the massage. The spot at the top of the jawbone under the ear lobes is an acupressure point called *vidhur* in Ayurveda, and it is renowned for helping with ear problems as well as jaw issues.

> **Weekly wellness hack** Each day this week reach out to a friend or family member you haven't spoken to for a while or who you don't speak to enough and who brings you joy. It can be a call, a message or even a little handwritten card to say "Hi". Human connection will boost your mood, feed your soul and help you feel supported and loved.

My Positive Word for the Week:

....

The Way I Want to Feel this Week:

....

My Reason for Doing Face Yoga this Week:

....

"You are not alone."

MONDAY

Today's intention:

....

When I did my Face Yoga today:

AM practice .... minutes   PM practice .... minutes

The areas I worked on today:

☐ Forehead ☐ Eyes ☐ Cheeks ☐ Mouth ☐ Jaw ☐ Neck ☐ Wellness

What I am most grateful for today:

....

....

TUESDAY

Today's intention:

....

When I did my Face Yoga today:

AM practice .... minutes   PM practice .... minutes

The areas I worked on today:

☐ Forehead ☐ Eyes ☐ Cheeks ☐ Mouth ☐ Jaw ☐ Neck ☐ Wellness

What I am most grateful for today:

....

....

WEDNESDAY

Today's intention:

....

When I did my Face Yoga today:

AM practice .... minutes   PM practice .... minutes

The areas I worked on today:

☐ Forehead ☐ Eyes ☐ Cheeks ☐ Mouth ☐ Jaw ☐ Neck ☐ Wellness

What I am most grateful for today:

....

....

THURSDAY

Today's intention:

....

When I did my Face Yoga today:

AM practice .... minutes   PM practice .... minutes

The areas I worked on today:

☐ Forehead ☐ Eyes ☐ Cheeks ☐ Mouth ☐ Jaw ☐ Neck ☐ Wellness

What I am most grateful for today:

....

....

FRIDAY

Today's intention:

....

When I did my Face Yoga today:

AM practice .... minutes   PM practice .... minutes

The areas I worked on today:

☐ Forehead ☐ Eyes ☐ Cheeks ☐ Mouth ☐ Jaw ☐ Neck ☐ Wellness

What I am most grateful for today:

....

....

SATURDAY

Today's intention:

....

When I did my Face Yoga today:

AM practice .... minutes   PM practice .... minutes

The areas I worked on today:

☐ Forehead ☐ Eyes ☐ Cheeks ☐ Mouth ☐ Jaw ☐ Neck ☐ Wellness

What I am most grateful for today:

....

....

SUNDAY

Today's intention:

....

When I did my Face Yoga today:

AM practice .... minutes   PM practice .... minutes

The areas I worked on today:

☐ Forehead ☐ Eyes ☐ Cheeks ☐ Mouth ☐ Jaw ☐ Neck ☐ Wellness

What I am most grateful for today:

....

....

What Went Well this Week:

....

....

What Didn't Go so Well this Week:

....

....

Week 7. Devotion

You have already devoted yourself to six weeks of wellness and Face Yoga, so the first thing to do this week is to celebrate that! Keep this thought in mind as you do your practices. Devoting yourself to this journal is a commitment, but each day this week, remember that it is well worth it and know that by now, you have formed habits which will last a lifetime.

TECHNIQUE OF THE WEEK
The Neck Devoting Technique

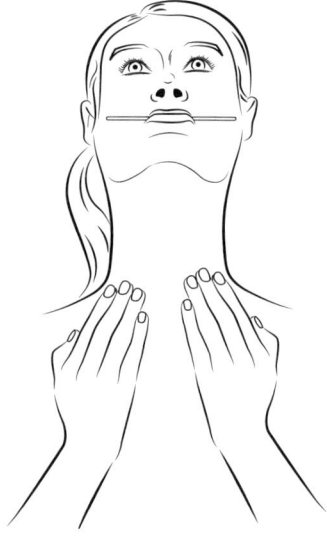

1. Slightly stick your bottom lip out and place a clean pencil between your lips. Gently tilt your head back as far as is comfortable, placing your fingertips on your collarbone for support and resistance. Use the strength of your mouth to hold the pencil in place for 30 seconds.

2. Relax completely then do this a second time for 30 seconds.

Benefits: This technique strengthens the platysma muscle at the front of the neck. As the muscle becomes more toned, the skin attached becomes firmer. This technique also helps to tone the muscles surrounding the lips to smooth lines in that area. Using a pencil is a great way to ensure both sides of the face are working in unison and balancing the pencil in place encourages the neck to stay engaged.

> **Weekly wellness hack** Each evening this week, eat your last meal by 7pm and then don't eat again until 7am the next morning. This will give your body a break from digesting food, which gives it the chance to focus on repairing and refreshing the skin and other organs.

My Positive Word for the Week:

....

The Way I Want to Feel this Week:

....

My Reason for Doing Face Yoga this Week:

....

"You will never regret devoting yourself to your own happiness."

MONDAY

Today's intention:

....

When I did my Face Yoga today:

AM practice .... minutes   PM practice .... minutes

The areas I worked on today:

☐ Forehead   ☐ Eyes   ☐ Cheeks   ☐ Mouth   ☐ Jaw   ☐ Neck   ☐ Wellness

What I am most grateful for today:

....

....

TUESDAY

Today's intention:

....

When I did my Face Yoga today:

AM practice .... minutes   PM practice .... minutes

The areas I worked on today:

☐ Forehead   ☐ Eyes   ☐ Cheeks   ☐ Mouth   ☐ Jaw   ☐ Neck   ☐ Wellness

What I am most grateful for today:

....

....

WEDNESDAY

Today's intention:

....

When I did my Face Yoga today:

AM practice .... minutes   PM practice .... minutes

The areas I worked on today:

☐ Forehead ☐ Eyes ☐ Cheeks ☐ Mouth ☐ Jaw ☐ Neck ☐ Wellness

What I am most grateful for today:

....

....

THURSDAY

Today's intention:

....

When I did my Face Yoga today:

AM practice .... minutes   PM practice .... minutes

The areas I worked on today:

☐ Forehead ☐ Eyes ☐ Cheeks ☐ Mouth ☐ Jaw ☐ Neck ☐ Wellness

What I am most grateful for today:

....

....

FRIDAY

Today's intention:

....

When I did my Face Yoga today:

AM practice .... minutes   PM practice .... minutes

The areas I worked on today:

☐ Forehead ☐ Eyes ☐ Cheeks ☐ Mouth ☐ Jaw ☐ Neck ☐ Wellness

What I am most grateful for today:

....

....

SATURDAY

Today's intention:

....

When I did my Face Yoga today:

AM practice .... minutes   PM practice .... minutes

The areas I worked on today:

☐ Forehead ☐ Eyes ☐ Cheeks ☐ Mouth ☐ Jaw ☐ Neck ☐ Wellness

What I am most grateful for today:

....

....

SUNDAY

Today's intention:

....

When I did my Face Yoga today:

AM practice .... minutes   PM practice .... minutes

The areas I worked on today:

☐ Forehead ☐ Eyes ☐ Cheeks ☐ Mouth ☐ Jaw ☐ Neck ☐ Wellness

What I am most grateful for today:

....

....

What Went Well this Week:

....

....

What Didn't Go so Well this Week:

....

....

Week 8. Grounding

Feeling grounded is about being settled, at peace and in tune with yourself and the environment around you. Your Face Yoga this week will help promote this feeling, as will your wellness hack. This week, aim to be really aware of what helps you feel grounded in your daily life (and what doesn't).

TECHNIQUE OF THE WEEK
The Forehead Grounding Technique

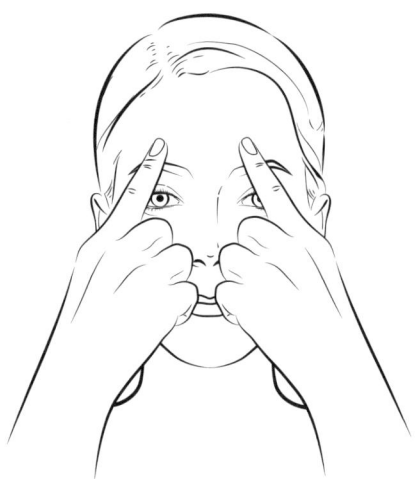

1. Place your two index fingers together between your eyebrows. Gently move them away from each other while making little semicircles in a line above your eyebrows. When you get to the outer edges of your eyebrows, lift your fingers off and move them to the middle of your forehead, making the same pattern out toward your hairline. Then do the same near the top of your forehead.

2. Repeat the whole sequence twice more.

Benefits: This technique helps to relax and soften your frontalis muscle in the forehead and prevents stress-related expression lines. It also helps this area to look more glowing by boosting circulation. It has the wellness benefit of stimulating acupressure points on the forehead which can help you to feel calm and grounded, and may even reduce headaches.

> **Weekly wellness hack** Every day this week, take some time, ideally alone, to be around nature. Look at the sky, look at the trees, the plants and the flowers. Let yourself be in awe of simple things like the pattern on a leaf or the shape of a cloud. This is super simple but so grounding for the mind, body and soul.

My Positive Word for the Week:

....

The Way I Want to Feel this Week:

....

My Reason for Doing Face Yoga this Week:

....

"Being a grounded person isn't about always being positive. It's about knowing there will be bad days, but good days are coming."

MONDAY

Today's intention:

....

When I did my Face Yoga today:

AM practice .... minutes   PM practice .... minutes

The areas I worked on today:

☐ Forehead ☐ Eyes ☐ Cheeks ☐ Mouth ☐ Jaw ☐ Neck ☐ Wellness

What I am most grateful for today:

....

....

TUESDAY

Today's intention:

....

When I did my Face Yoga today:

AM practice .... minutes   PM practice .... minutes

The areas I worked on today:

☐ Forehead ☐ Eyes ☐ Cheeks ☐ Mouth ☐ Jaw ☐ Neck ☐ Wellness

What I am most grateful for today:

....

....

WEDNESDAY

Today's intention:

....

When I did my Face Yoga today:

AM practice .... minutes   PM practice .... minutes

The areas I worked on today:

☐ Forehead ☐ Eyes ☐ Cheeks ☐ Mouth ☐ Jaw ☐ Neck ☐ Wellness

What I am most grateful for today:

....

....

THURSDAY

Today's intention:

....

When I did my Face Yoga today:

AM practice .... minutes   PM practice .... minutes

The areas I worked on today:

☐ Forehead ☐ Eyes ☐ Cheeks ☐ Mouth ☐ Jaw ☐ Neck ☐ Wellness

What I am most grateful for today:

....

....

FRIDAY

Today's intention:

....

When I did my Face Yoga today:

AM practice .... minutes   PM practice .... minutes

The areas I worked on today:

☐ Forehead ☐ Eyes ☐ Cheeks ☐ Mouth ☐ Jaw ☐ Neck ☐ Wellness

What I am most grateful for today:

....

....

SATURDAY

Today's intention:

....

When I did my Face Yoga today:

AM practice .... minutes   PM practice .... minutes

The areas I worked on today:

☐ Forehead ☐ Eyes ☐ Cheeks ☐ Mouth ☐ Jaw ☐ Neck ☐ Wellness

What I am most grateful for today:

....

....

SUNDAY

Today's intention:

....

When I did my Face Yoga today:

AM practice .... minutes   PM practice .... minutes

The areas I worked on today:

☐ Forehead ☐ Eyes ☐ Cheeks ☐ Mouth ☐ Jaw ☐ Neck ☐ Wellness

What I am most grateful for today:

....

....

What Went Well this Week:

....

....

What Didn't Go so Well this Week:

....

....

Week 9. Shining

This week is about shining inside and out. Your Face Yoga technique helps the eyes to gleam and look and feel alive, and your wellness hack is a powerful way of maintaining inner shine as well as radiating out this glowing energy. Another great way to shine from the inside out this week is to revisit your yellow topaz crystals and the colour yellow and think about how you can incorporate these into your routine.

TECHNIQUE OF THE WEEK
The Eye Shining Technique

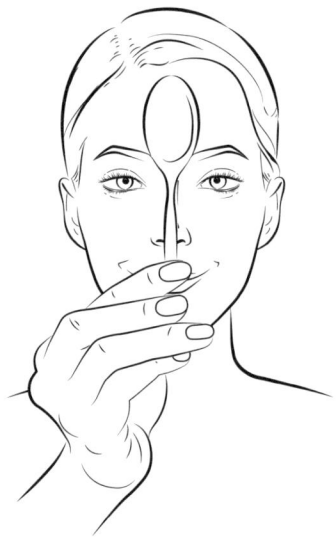

1. Hold a teaspoon out in front of your face at arm's length. Move it around in a large figure of 8. Keep your eyes fixed on the teaspoon but don't move your head or the rest of your face.

2. After 30 seconds, move the teaspoon in the other direction.

Benefits: This exercises the eye muscles. As the muscles surrounding your eye become stronger and more toned, the skin attached becomes smoother, helping to soften and reduce fine lines. It also helps to reinvigorate fatigued eyes and gives them a healthy shine.

> **Weekly wellness hack** Any time you feel fatigued, sad or around people that you feel uncomfortable with, try visualizing a shining, beautiful yellow light surrounding your body and face. Imagine this protects your energy as well as allows you to radiate positive vibes to the people you meet.

My Positive Word for the Week:

....

The Way I Want to Feel this Week:

....

My Reason for Doing Face Yoga this Week:

....

"Remember it's not your job to prove your worthiness to anyone."

MONDAY

Today's intention:

....

When I did my Face Yoga today:

AM practice .... minutes   PM practice .... minutes

The areas I worked on today:

☐ Forehead ☐ Eyes ☐ Cheeks ☐ Mouth ☐ Jaw ☐ Neck ☐ Wellness

What I am most grateful for today:

....

....

TUESDAY

Today's intention:

....

When I did my Face Yoga today:

AM practice .... minutes   PM practice .... minutes

The areas I worked on today:

☐ Forehead ☐ Eyes ☐ Cheeks ☐ Mouth ☐ Jaw ☐ Neck ☐ Wellness

What I am most grateful for today:

....

....

WEDNESDAY

Today's intention:

....

When I did my Face Yoga today:

AM practice .... minutes   PM practice .... minutes

The areas I worked on today:

☐ Forehead ☐ Eyes ☐ Cheeks ☐ Mouth ☐ Jaw ☐ Neck ☐ Wellness

What I am most grateful for today:

....

....

THURSDAY

Today's intention:

....

When I did my Face Yoga today:

AM practice .... minutes   PM practice .... minutes

The areas I worked on today:

☐ Forehead ☐ Eyes ☐ Cheeks ☐ Mouth ☐ Jaw ☐ Neck ☐ Wellness

What I am most grateful for today:

....

....

FRIDAY

Today's intention:

....

When I did my Face Yoga today:

AM practice .... minutes   PM practice .... minutes

The areas I worked on today:

☐ Forehead ☐ Eyes ☐ Cheeks ☐ Mouth ☐ Jaw ☐ Neck ☐ Wellness

What I am most grateful for today:

....

....

SATURDAY

Today's intention:

....

When I did my Face Yoga today:

AM practice .... minutes   PM practice .... minutes

The areas I worked on today:

☐ Forehead ☐ Eyes ☐ Cheeks ☐ Mouth ☐ Jaw ☐ Neck ☐ Wellness

What I am most grateful for today:

....

....

SUNDAY

Today's intention:

....

When I did my Face Yoga today:

AM practice .... minutes   PM practice .... minutes

The areas I worked on today:

☐ Forehead   ☐ Eyes   ☐ Cheeks   ☐ Mouth   ☐ Jaw   ☐ Neck   ☐ Wellness

What I am most grateful for today:

....

....

What Went Well this Week:

....

....

What Didn't Go so Well this Week:

....

....

Week 10. Enlivening

Our busy, fast-paced lives mean it can be easy to forget to enliven the joy within us. We can often take everything so seriously, forgetting that life is short and happiness and fun need to be part of our day, every day. When we enliven the joy within us, we can see a shift. We get less stressed about the small things, we see the humour in many situations and we ignite our passion for the things we love.

TECHNIQUE OF THE WEEK
The Cheek Enlivening Technique

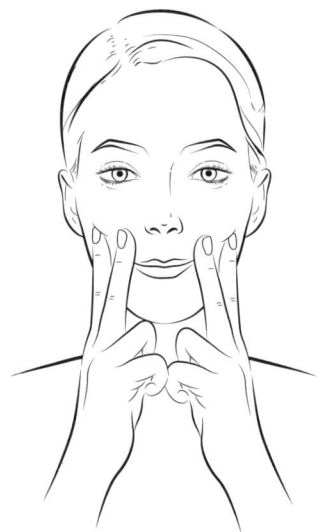

1. Using both hands, place your index and middle fingers directly below your mouth corners, just above your jawbone. With a little serum on the skin, start to glide your fingers upward, separating your middle and index fingers away from each other so they form a "V" shape.

2. Stop when your middle fingers reach just above your nostrils and lift off. Repeat and keep this going for 1 minute.

Benefits: This helps your cheeks to look enlivened by boosting the circulation. It also releases tension from this area, helping to soften lines such as the nasolabial folds between the nostrils and the corners of the mouth and marionette lines below the corners of the mouth, which are often caused by repetitive stress-related expressions. It also encourages your muscles to become toned.

> **Weekly wellness hack** Each day this week wear something special and notice how it enlivens your mind, body and soul. It may be a nice dress, a special piece of jewellery or a pair of high heels. Try to wear something green to balance your heart chakra. This is about reminding yourself that being alive and well needs to be celebrated and you deserve to look and feel your very best – and to give yourself some love!

My Positive Word for the Week:

....

The Way I Want to Feel this Week:

....

My Reason for Doing Face Yoga this Week:

....

"Stop saving things for a special occasion. Life is short, being here today is the special occasion."

MONDAY

Today's intention:

....

When I did my Face Yoga today:

AM practice .... minutes   PM practice .... minutes

The areas I worked on today:

☐ Forehead ☐ Eyes ☐ Cheeks ☐ Mouth ☐ Jaw ☐ Neck ☐ Wellness

What I am most grateful for today:

....

....

TUESDAY

Today's intention:

....

When I did my Face Yoga today:

AM practice .... minutes   PM practice .... minutes

The areas I worked on today:

☐ Forehead ☐ Eyes ☐ Cheeks ☐ Mouth ☐ Jaw ☐ Neck ☐ Wellness

What I am most grateful for today:

....

....

WEDNESDAY

Today's intention:

....

When I did my Face Yoga today:

AM practice .... minutes   PM practice .... minutes

The areas I worked on today:

☐ Forehead ☐ Eyes ☐ Cheeks ☐ Mouth ☐ Jaw ☐ Neck ☐ Wellness

What I am most grateful for today:

....

....

THURSDAY

Today's intention:

....

When I did my Face Yoga today:

AM practice .... minutes   PM practice .... minutes

The areas I worked on today:

☐ Forehead ☐ Eyes ☐ Cheeks ☐ Mouth ☐ Jaw ☐ Neck ☐ Wellness

What I am most grateful for today:

....

....

FRIDAY

Today's intention:

....

When I did my Face Yoga today:

AM practice .... minutes   PM practice .... minutes

The areas I worked on today:

☐ Forehead   ☐ Eyes   ☐ Cheeks   ☐ Mouth   ☐ Jaw   ☐ Neck   ☐ Wellness

What I am most grateful for today:

....

....

SATURDAY

Today's intention:

....

When I did my Face Yoga today:

AM practice .... minutes   PM practice .... minutes

The areas I worked on today:

☐ Forehead   ☐ Eyes   ☐ Cheeks   ☐ Mouth   ☐ Jaw   ☐ Neck   ☐ Wellness

What I am most grateful for today:

....

....

SUNDAY

Today's intention:

....

When I did my Face Yoga today:

AM practice .... minutes   PM practice .... minutes

The areas I worked on today:

☐ Forehead ☐ Eyes ☐ Cheeks ☐ Mouth ☐ Jaw ☐ Neck ☐ Wellness

What I am most grateful for today:

....

....

What Went Well this Week:

....

....

What Didn't Go so Well this Week:

....

....

Week 11. Adoration

You deserve to be adored, by yourself and by others. This season is focused on love, and adoration is a huge part of that. As you go through your week, look at ways that you can adore yourself (your Face Yoga practice is one way, of course) and how you can also adore qualities in others. This will boost your oxytocin and balance your heart chakra, which helps with self-love as well as receiving love from others.

The Mouth Adoring Technique

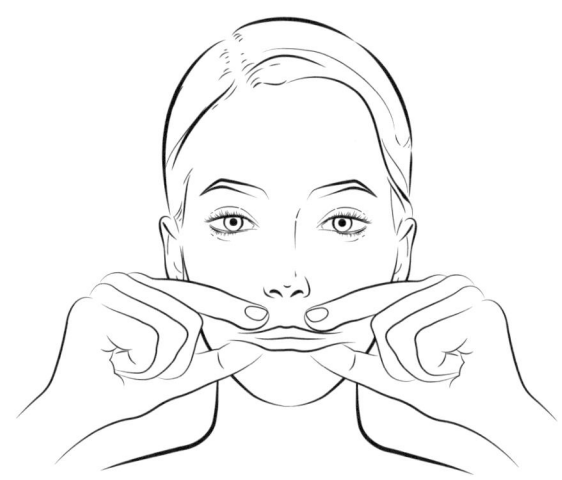

1. Start with your lips gently closed. Place your index fingers above your top lip and thumbs below your bottom lip and start to squeeze the lips together so they form a straight line. Hold for 20 seconds.

2. Gently release and do twice more.

Benefits: This helps to boost the circulation to the circular muscle around the lips. It's great to do if you are prone to small lines around the lips or to nasolabial folds between the nostrils and the corners of the mouth.

Weekly wellness hack Do a daily "self-adoration" dance. This may feel very much out of your comfort zone but please try! Every day, play two songs which make you feel really great, find a space on your own and dance in any way your body wants to move. Feel the adoration, love and release of this practice.

My Positive Word for the Week:

....

The Way I Want to Feel this Week:

....

My Reason for Doing Face Yoga this Week:

....

"Choose love over fear."

MONDAY

Today's intention:

....

When I did my Face Yoga today:

AM practice .... minutes   PM practice .... minutes

The areas I worked on today:

☐ Forehead ☐ Eyes ☐ Cheeks ☐ Mouth ☐ Jaw ☐ Neck ☐ Wellness

What I am most grateful for today:

....

....

TUESDAY

Today's intention:

....

When I did my Face Yoga today:

AM practice .... minutes   PM practice .... minutes

The areas I worked on today:

☐ Forehead ☐ Eyes ☐ Cheeks ☐ Mouth ☐ Jaw ☐ Neck ☐ Wellness

What I am most grateful for today:

....

....

WEDNESDAY

Today's intention:

....

When I did my Face Yoga today:

AM practice .... minutes   PM practice .... minutes

The areas I worked on today:

☐ Forehead ☐ Eyes ☐ Cheeks ☐ Mouth ☐ Jaw ☐ Neck ☐ Wellness

What I am most grateful for today:

....

....

THURSDAY

Today's intention:

....

When I did my Face Yoga today:

AM practice .... minutes   PM practice .... minutes

The areas I worked on today:

☐ Forehead ☐ Eyes ☐ Cheeks ☐ Mouth ☐ Jaw ☐ Neck ☐ Wellness

What I am most grateful for today:

....

....

FRIDAY

Today's intention:

....

When I did my Face Yoga today:

AM practice .... minutes   PM practice .... minutes

The areas I worked on today:

☐ Forehead   ☐ Eyes   ☐ Cheeks   ☐ Mouth   ☐ Jaw   ☐ Neck   ☐ Wellness

What I am most grateful for today:

....

....

SATURDAY

Today's intention:

....

When I did my Face Yoga today:

AM practice .... minutes   PM practice .... minutes

The areas I worked on today:

☐ Forehead   ☐ Eyes   ☐ Cheeks   ☐ Mouth   ☐ Jaw   ☐ Neck   ☐ Wellness

What I am most grateful for today:

....

....

SUNDAY

Today's intention:

....

When I did my Face Yoga today:

AM practice .... minutes   PM practice .... minutes

The areas I worked on today:

☐ Forehead ☐ Eyes ☐ Cheeks ☐ Mouth ☐ Jaw ☐ Neck ☐ Wellness

What I am most grateful for today:

....

....

What Went Well this Week:

....

....

What Didn't Go so Well this Week:

....

....

Week 12. Warmth

The Danish concept of *hygge* is what I want you to focus on this week, whatever the weather. Hygge is about cosiness, warmth and spending time feeling relaxed, at peace and at ease. It can be created through external sources such as blankets and candles; however, it's not just about things but more about internal warmth, self-care and self-love. As you do your Face Yoga, your wellness hack and gratitude practice this week, have this thought in mind.

TECHNIQUE OF THE WEEK
The Jaw Warming Technique

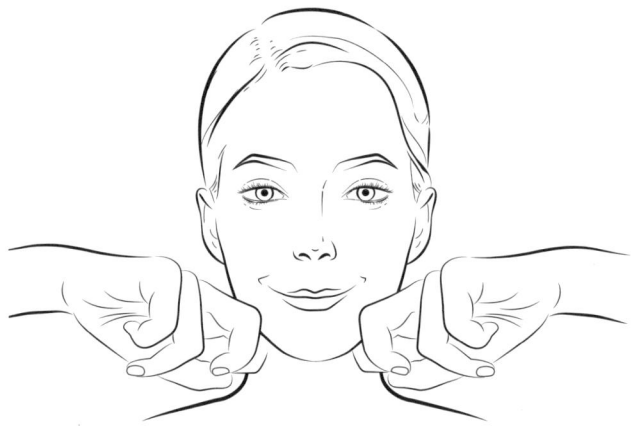

1. Using both hands, place the joints of your index and middle fingers together in the centre of your chin. Glide your hands away from each other toward your ears, so the joints of your middle fingers move above your jawbone and the joints of your index fingers move below it.

2. When the joints of your index fingers are nestled under the ear lobes at the top of the jawbone, lift off and start again.

3. Continue the massage for 1 minute.

Benefits: This helps to ease mental and physical stress that can manifest in the jaw muscle, as well as encouraging the muscles to lift upward. You will feel a warmth in the lower face after you complete it, as you will have increased your *chi* or *prana*, which is your subtle energy. This means the lower face will look and feel healthier.

> **Weekly wellness hack** Enjoy the warming power of touch. Spend more time than usual hugging or stroking your pet, partner or children. Or if you live alone, get some massage oil and massage your own arms and legs. Try to really feel connected to your own skin. Touch is so powerful for your mental and physical wellbeing.

My Positive Word for the Week:

....

The Way I Want to Feel this Week:

....

My Reason for Doing Face Yoga this Week:

....

"Spend time with people who warm your heart."

MONDAY

Today's intention:

....

When I did my Face Yoga today:

AM practice .... minutes   PM practice .... minutes

The areas I worked on today:

☐ Forehead ☐ Eyes ☐ Cheeks ☐ Mouth ☐ Jaw ☐ Neck ☐ Wellness

What I am most grateful for today:

....

....

TUESDAY

Today's intention:

....

When I did my Face Yoga today:

AM practice .... minutes   PM practice .... minutes

The areas I worked on today:

☐ Forehead ☐ Eyes ☐ Cheeks ☐ Mouth ☐ Jaw ☐ Neck ☐ Wellness

What I am most grateful for today:

....

....

WEDNESDAY

Today's intention:

....

When I did my Face Yoga today:

AM practice .... minutes   PM practice .... minutes

The areas I worked on today:

☐ Forehead ☐ Eyes ☐ Cheeks ☐ Mouth ☐ Jaw ☐ Neck ☐ Wellness

What I am most grateful for today:

....

....

THURSDAY

Today's intention:

....

When I did my Face Yoga today:

AM practice .... minutes   PM practice .... minutes

The areas I worked on today:

☐ Forehead ☐ Eyes ☐ Cheeks ☐ Mouth ☐ Jaw ☐ Neck ☐ Wellness

What I am most grateful for today:

....

....

FRIDAY

Today's intention:

....

When I did my Face Yoga today:

AM practice .... minutes   PM practice .... minutes

The areas I worked on today:

☐ Forehead ☐ Eyes ☐ Cheeks ☐ Mouth ☐ Jaw ☐ Neck ☐ Wellness

What I am most grateful for today:

....

....

SATURDAY

Today's intention:

....

When I did my Face Yoga today:

AM practice .... minutes   PM practice .... minutes

The areas I worked on today:

☐ Forehead ☐ Eyes ☐ Cheeks ☐ Mouth ☐ Jaw ☐ Neck ☐ Wellness

What I am most grateful for today:

....

....

SUNDAY

Today's intention:

....

When I did my Face Yoga today:

AM practice .... minutes   PM practice .... minutes

The areas I worked on today:

☐ Forehead ☐ Eyes ☐ Cheeks ☐ Mouth ☐ Jaw ☐ Neck ☐ Wellness

What I am most grateful for today:

....

....

What Went Well this Week:

....

....

What Didn't Go so Well this Week:

....

....

Week 13. Care

Self-care and care for others both have an important place when it comes to your mental and physical wellness. The key is finding a balance. Great wellness comes from extending kindness to the people in your lives as often as you can whilst maintaining your own energy through self-care. Your Face Yoga this week is gentle yet powerful, so do it anytime you feel the need to care for yourself mentally and physically.

TECHNIQUE OF THE WEEK
The Neck Caring Technique

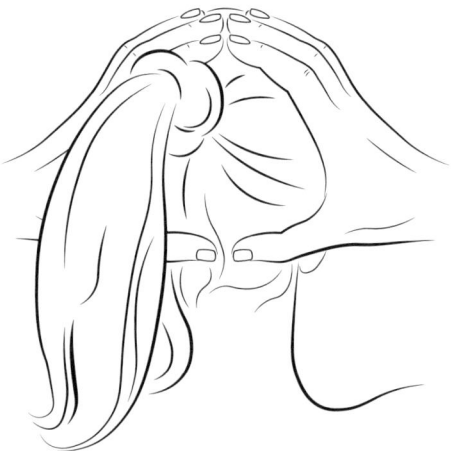

1. Place your two thumbs next to each other at the base of your skull and cup the hands lightly over the back of your head. Massage this point in a clockwise circular motion about 5 times, then move the thumbs slightly away from each other and massage on another point, gradually and intuitively working along the occipital bone/base of the skull until you reach the ears.

2. Lift off and repeat again but this time massage in an anticlockwise direction. The whole sequence should take around 1 minute.

Benefits: This directly eases tension at the back of the head and indirectly reduces strain in the face, because when your head and neck are relaxed, your facial muscles can relax too. It's also a wonderful way to care for the mind as stress dissipates.

> **Weekly wellness hack** As many times as you can this week, have a ritual bath. Run a warm bath, place some candles and crystals (perhaps rose quartz and yellow topaz) around the bath and sprinkle in bath oils, salts or even a few flower petals. Turn down the lights and remind yourself that you deserve self-care.

My Positive Word for the Week:

....

The Way I Want to Feel this Week:

....

My Reason for Doing Face Yoga this Week:

....

"Maybe it's not working out because something better is on its way for you."

MONDAY

Today's intention:

....

When I did my Face Yoga today:

AM practice .... minutes   PM practice .... minutes

The areas I worked on today:

☐ Forehead ☐ Eyes ☐ Cheeks ☐ Mouth ☐ Jaw ☐ Neck ☐ Wellness

What I am most grateful for today:

....

....

TUESDAY

Today's intention:

....

When I did my Face Yoga today:

AM practice .... minutes   PM practice .... minutes

The areas I worked on today:

☐ Forehead ☐ Eyes ☐ Cheeks ☐ Mouth ☐ Jaw ☐ Neck ☐ Wellness

What I am most grateful for today:

....

....

WEDNESDAY

Today's intention:

....

When I did my Face Yoga today:

AM practice .... minutes   PM practice .... minutes

The areas I worked on today:

☐ Forehead ☐ Eyes ☐ Cheeks ☐ Mouth ☐ Jaw ☐ Neck ☐ Wellness

What I am most grateful for today:

....

....

THURSDAY

Today's intention:

....

When I did my Face Yoga today:

AM practice .... minutes   PM practice .... minutes

The areas I worked on today:

☐ Forehead ☐ Eyes ☐ Cheeks ☐ Mouth ☐ Jaw ☐ Neck ☐ Wellness

What I am most grateful for today:

....

....

FRIDAY

Today's intention:

....

When I did my Face Yoga today:

AM practice .... minutes   PM practice .... minutes

The areas I worked on today:

☐ Forehead   ☐ Eyes   ☐ Cheeks   ☐ Mouth   ☐ Jaw   ☐ Neck   ☐ Wellness

What I am most grateful for today:

....

....

SATURDAY

Today's intention:

....

When I did my Face Yoga today:

AM practice .... minutes   PM practice .... minutes

The areas I worked on today:

☐ Forehead   ☐ Eyes   ☐ Cheeks   ☐ Mouth   ☐ Jaw   ☐ Neck   ☐ Wellness

What I am most grateful for today:

....

....

SUNDAY

Today's intention:

....

When I did my Face Yoga today:

AM practice .... minutes   PM practice .... minutes

The areas I worked on today:

☐ Forehead ☐ Eyes ☐ Cheeks ☐ Mouth ☐ Jaw ☐ Neck ☐ Wellness

What I am most grateful for today:

....

....

What Went Well this Week:

....

....

What Didn't Go so Well this Week:

....

....

Season 2
Energize your face

Happiness chemical: endorphins
Chakras: crown chakra and sacral chakra
Crystals: clear quartz and sunstone
Colours: white (or pale purple) and orange

Mantra: "I know and understand that I deserve to feel great."

Everything is energy. The word energy has so many meanings and interpretations. This season, we are going to focus on energy in two ways. Firstly, we are going to increase vitality and vigour. Your Face Yoga techniques for the next 13 weeks are designed to help your skin look energized, and also ease fatigue and dullness so you *feel* energized too. One of the things I have noted during my years as The Face Yoga Expert is that energized skin is truly what makes us look youthful, even more so than how many lines or wrinkles we have or don't have.

Secondly, we are focusing on energy in the yogic sense of *prana* and *chi* or *qi* in Traditional Chinese Medicine, which all mean "life force" or "vital energy" and which flow through every living thing. To help unlock your *prana* or *chi* and to allow it to flow freely throughout the face, mind and body, my first recommendation would be to focus on deep breathing daily, particularly during your Face Yoga practice. Doing activities which make you feel good (boost endorphins) help energy in both senses of the word too.

Focusing on the crown chakra, which can be done through surrounding yourself with the colour white (or pale purple) and using a clear quartz crystal, helps you connect to your energy at the highest level, which is your consciousness and inner wisdom. The sacral chakra is the energy centre to awaken and balance emotions, so using a sunstone and the colour orange is another great way to boost energy and energies. Your mantra is a combination of words which connect to both chakras and is designed to help your life energy flow freely.

All the weekly themes are designed to help your skin look and feel energized. They help to bring vitality to the face, energy to the mind and wake up your body, too.

Week 14. Refreshing

This week is about looking and feeling refreshed. It's a great place to start a new season that is focused on energy. As you write your positive word, the way you want to feel and your reason for doing Face Yoga this week, think about what areas of your life, mind, body and face need a refresh, rebirth and new energy.

TECHNIQUE OF THE WEEK

The Face Refreshing Technique

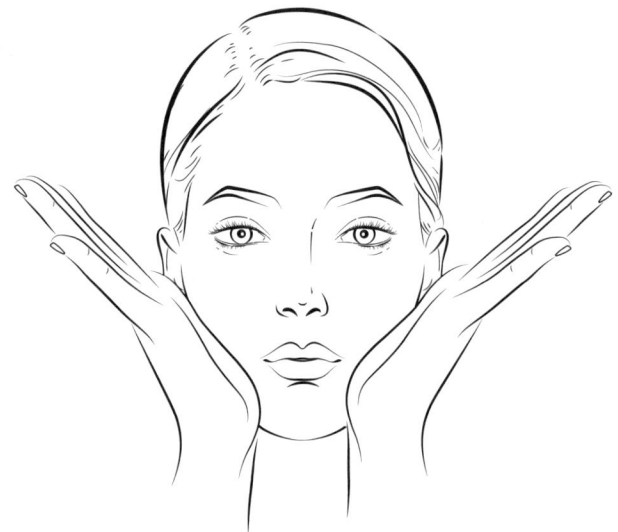

1. Place the base of your thumbs on the jaw muscle, just below the mouth. Making sure you have serum or oil on the skin, gently massage in little circles up the jaw on both sides of your face. Then massage over your cheeks, up to your temples and then along your forehead until your thumbs meet in the middle of the forehead.

2. Repeat the sequence twice more.

Benefits: This full-face massage helps your skin to look and feel more refreshed by boosting the blood flow and easing tension. It also helps your serum penetrate deeper into the skin, so it can reach the middle layer of skin or dermis where your collagen and elastin lie. This can help refresh, plump and firm the skin by regenerating new skin cells.

Weekly wellness hack Once a day this week, try this qigong technique. Start by shaking your hands, then your arms, then move to your feet and your legs. Then shake your whole body. Notice how refreshed and energized you instantly feel.

My Positive Word for the Week:

....

The Way I Want to Feel this Week:

....

My Reason for Doing Face Yoga this Week:

....

"The easiest way to refresh your mind and body is to start giving more energy to the things that give you energy."

MONDAY

Today's intention:

....

When I did my Face Yoga today:

AM practice .... minutes   PM practice .... minutes

The areas I worked on today:

☐ Forehead   ☐ Eyes   ☐ Cheeks   ☐ Mouth   ☐ Jaw   ☐ Neck   ☐ Wellness

What I am most grateful for today:

....

....

TUESDAY

Today's intention:

....

When I did my Face Yoga today:

AM practice .... minutes   PM practice .... minutes

The areas I worked on today:

☐ Forehead   ☐ Eyes   ☐ Cheeks   ☐ Mouth   ☐ Jaw   ☐ Neck   ☐ Wellness

What I am most grateful for today:

....

....

WEDNESDAY

Today's intention:

....

When I did my Face Yoga today:

AM practice .... minutes   PM practice .... minutes

The areas I worked on today:

☐ Forehead ☐ Eyes ☐ Cheeks ☐ Mouth ☐ Jaw ☐ Neck ☐ Wellness

What I am most grateful for today:

....

....

THURSDAY

Today's intention:

....

When I did my Face Yoga today:

AM practice .... minutes   PM practice .... minutes

The areas I worked on today:

☐ Forehead ☐ Eyes ☐ Cheeks ☐ Mouth ☐ Jaw ☐ Neck ☐ Wellness

What I am most grateful for today:

....

....

FRIDAY

Today's intention:

....

When I did my Face Yoga today:

AM practice .... minutes   PM practice .... minutes

The areas I worked on today:

☐ Forehead ☐ Eyes ☐ Cheeks ☐ Mouth ☐ Jaw ☐ Neck ☐ Wellness

What I am most grateful for today:

....

....

SATURDAY

Today's intention:

....

When I did my Face Yoga today:

AM practice .... minutes   PM practice .... minutes

The areas I worked on today:

☐ Forehead ☐ Eyes ☐ Cheeks ☐ Mouth ☐ Jaw ☐ Neck ☐ Wellness

What I am most grateful for today:

....

....

SUNDAY

Today's intention:

....

When I did my Face Yoga today:

AM practice .... minutes   PM practice .... minutes

The areas I worked on today:

☐ Forehead ☐ Eyes ☐ Cheeks ☐ Mouth ☐ Jaw ☐ Neck ☐ Wellness

What I am most grateful for today:

....

....

What Went Well this Week:

....

....

What Didn't Go so Well this Week:

....

....

Week 15. Rejuvenation

This week is about doing what your face, body and mind need in order to rejuvenate. When your energy is low, stuck or out of balance, your forehead area and eyebrows tend to tense and even droop, your mind feels overwhelmed and your body tired. This week, between your Face Yoga technique, your wellness hack and your positive statement, you have some simple tools to rejuvenate. Wearing orange to balance your sacral chakra (the centre of your feelings and sensations) is a great way to assist a week of rejuvenation.

TECHNIQUE OF THE WEEK
The Forehead Rejuvenating Technique

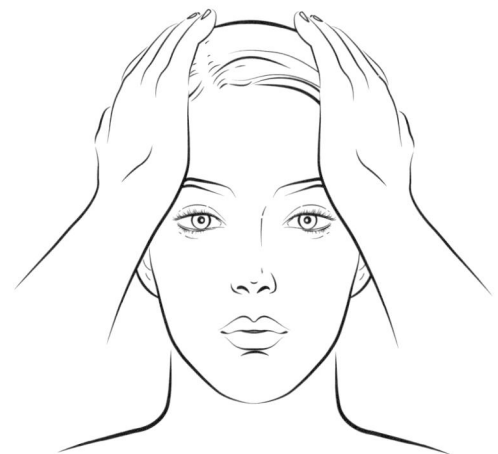

1. Place the heel of your hands over your eyebrows, gently lifting the outer third of the eyebrows only. Open your eyes wide to make sure you aren't creasing the skin on your forehead. Your fingers are lightly resting on the top of your head. Hold for 30 seconds, then lift off.

2. Repeat once more.

Benefits: This lifts sagging eyebrows, strengthens and opens up the eye area and eases head tension. It is great for helping the eyes look and feel more rejuvenated and energized.

> **Weekly wellness hack** Give yourself a moment each day to do nothing. No screens, no people, no distractions. Just sit and breathe with your eyes closed or look out a window or simply be still in your favourite outdoor space. Notice what feelings and emotions come up, both good and bad, and just sit with them for a few minutes. You will emerge feeling rejuvenated in mind, body and face.

My Positive Word for the Week:

....

The Way I Want to Feel this Week:

....

My Reason for Doing Face Yoga this Week:

....

"Rest. Rest as much as you need to until you are rejuvenated and ready to get going again. Just don't quit."

MONDAY

Today's intention:

....

When I did my Face Yoga today:

AM practice .... minutes   PM practice .... minutes

The areas I worked on today:

☐ Forehead ☐ Eyes ☐ Cheeks ☐ Mouth ☐ Jaw ☐ Neck ☐ Wellness

What I am most grateful for today:

....

....

TUESDAY

Today's intention:

....

When I did my Face Yoga today:

AM practice .... minutes   PM practice .... minutes

The areas I worked on today:

☐ Forehead ☐ Eyes ☐ Cheeks ☐ Mouth ☐ Jaw ☐ Neck ☐ Wellness

What I am most grateful for today:

....

....

WEDNESDAY

Today's intention:

....

When I did my Face Yoga today:

AM practice .... minutes   PM practice .... minutes

The areas I worked on today:

☐ Forehead ☐ Eyes ☐ Cheeks ☐ Mouth ☐ Jaw ☐ Neck ☐ Wellness

What I am most grateful for today:

....

....

THURSDAY

Today's intention:

....

When I did my Face Yoga today:

AM practice .... minutes   PM practice .... minutes

The areas I worked on today:

☐ Forehead ☐ Eyes ☐ Cheeks ☐ Mouth ☐ Jaw ☐ Neck ☐ Wellness

What I am most grateful for today:

....

....

FRIDAY

Today's intention:

....

When I did my Face Yoga today:

AM practice .... minutes   PM practice .... minutes

The areas I worked on today:

☐ Forehead   ☐ Eyes   ☐ Cheeks   ☐ Mouth   ☐ Jaw   ☐ Neck   ☐ Wellness

What I am most grateful for today:

....

....

SATURDAY

Today's intention:

....

When I did my Face Yoga today:

AM practice .... minutes   PM practice .... minutes

The areas I worked on today:

☐ Forehead   ☐ Eyes   ☐ Cheeks   ☐ Mouth   ☐ Jaw   ☐ Neck   ☐ Wellness

What I am most grateful for today:

....

....

SUNDAY

Today's intention:

....

When I did my Face Yoga today:

AM practice .... minutes   PM practice .... minutes

The areas I worked on today:

☐ Forehead ☐ Eyes ☐ Cheeks ☐ Mouth ☐ Jaw ☐ Neck ☐ Wellness

What I am most grateful for today:

....

....

What Went Well this Week:

....

....

What Didn't Go so Well this Week:

....

....

Week 16. Hydration

More than 60 per cent of the human body is made up of water, so in essence we are more water than anything else. Your mind and body need good hydration to work effectively and one of the most important things you can do for your skin is give it water through food and drink. When skin is dehydrated it has less plumpness and firmness (reduced skin turgor), lines and wrinkles are more visible and it can be flaky, inflamed and bloated. Hydrated skin looks younger, fresher and has fewer lines and wrinkles. The eyes can be prone to drying when they are tired and energy is stagnant.

TECHNIQUE OF THE WEEK
The Eye Hydrating Technique

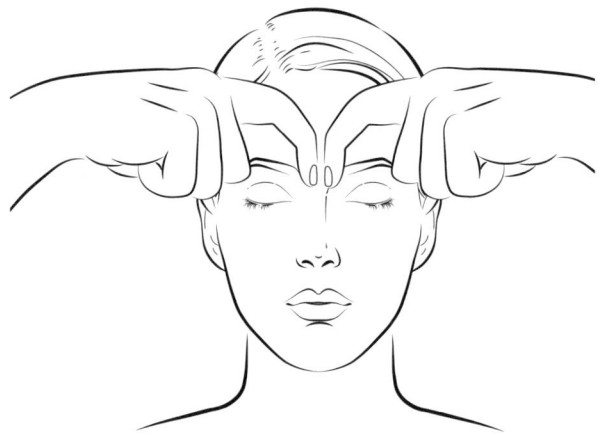

1. Form semicircles with your index fingers and place them above your eyebrows with the fingertips between your eyebrows. Rest the front of your thumbs (where the nail is) on the outer corners of the eyes, giving you support but also smoothing the skin. Close your eyes and slightly squeeze them so you feel a little shake or pulse. Hold for 30 seconds.

2. Relax and repeat once more.

Benefits: This is great for strengthening the muscles around the eye, particularly the outer corners, so it's really good for smoothing fine lines. It also helps to improve hydration to tired and dry eyes by increasing blood flow. When you move your eyes you naturally hydrate them with the fluid in your eyes. Dry eyes often come from not moving them or blinking enough.

> **Weekly wellness hack** Every day drink 2 litres of water (depending on what exercise you do and the weather, this may be more or slightly less) and be creative with your water. Try adding lemon, fresh mint or cucumber for some variation, flavour and nutrition.

My Positive Word for the Week:

....

The Way I Want to Feel this Week:

....

My Reason for Doing Face Yoga this Week:

....

"Ask your body every day: what do you need? Listen to the answer."

MONDAY

Today's intention:

....

When I did my Face Yoga today:

AM practice .... minutes   PM practice .... minutes

The areas I worked on today:

☐ Forehead   ☐ Eyes   ☐ Cheeks   ☐ Mouth   ☐ Jaw   ☐ Neck   ☐ Wellness

What I am most grateful for today:

....

....

TUESDAY

Today's intention:

....

When I did my Face Yoga today:

AM practice .... minutes   PM practice .... minutes

The areas I worked on today:

☐ Forehead   ☐ Eyes   ☐ Cheeks   ☐ Mouth   ☐ Jaw   ☐ Neck   ☐ Wellness

What I am most grateful for today:

....

....

WEDNESDAY

Today's intention:

....

When I did my Face Yoga today:

AM practice .... minutes   PM practice .... minutes

The areas I worked on today:

☐ Forehead ☐ Eyes ☐ Cheeks ☐ Mouth ☐ Jaw ☐ Neck ☐ Wellness

What I am most grateful for today:

....

....

THURSDAY

Today's intention:

....

When I did my Face Yoga today:

AM practice .... minutes   PM practice .... minutes

The areas I worked on today:

☐ Forehead ☐ Eyes ☐ Cheeks ☐ Mouth ☐ Jaw ☐ Neck ☐ Wellness

What I am most grateful for today:

....

....

FRIDAY

Today's intention:

....

When I did my Face Yoga today:

AM practice .... minutes   PM practice .... minutes

The areas I worked on today:

☐ Forehead ☐ Eyes ☐ Cheeks ☐ Mouth ☐ Jaw ☐ Neck ☐ Wellness

What I am most grateful for today:

....

....

SATURDAY

Today's intention:

....

When I did my Face Yoga today:

AM practice .... minutes   PM practice .... minutes

The areas I worked on today:

☐ Forehead ☐ Eyes ☐ Cheeks ☐ Mouth ☐ Jaw ☐ Neck ☐ Wellness

What I am most grateful for today:

....

....

SUNDAY

Today's intention:

....

When I did my Face Yoga today:

AM practice .... minutes   PM practice .... minutes

The areas I worked on today:

☐ Forehead ☐ Eyes ☐ Cheeks ☐ Mouth ☐ Jaw ☐ Neck ☐ Wellness

What I am most grateful for today:

....

....

What Went Well this Week:

....

....

What Didn't Go so Well this Week:

....

....

Week 17. Boosting

Your mantra for this season is about knowing and understanding that you deserve to feel great. Saying this to yourself will help boost your energy, mood, body and face and increase your endorphins. Adding in your wellness hack and reading this week's quote will further enhance this. This week your Face Yoga technique is a strong yet subtle movement aimed at boosting circulation and muscle tone.

TECHNIQUE OF THE WEEK
The Cheek Boosting Technique

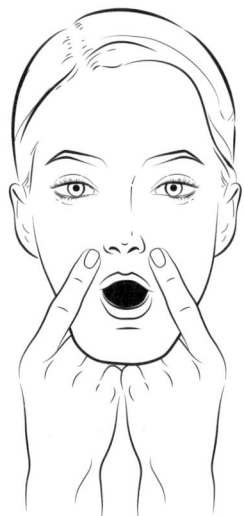

1. Make your mouth into a really small "O" shape with your lips slightly curled in. Place your index fingers on the line from your nostrils to your jawbone. Start lifting up the corners of your mouth into more of a smile.

2. Keep moving from the "O" to the small smile for 1 minute, using the index fingers to stop any lines forming and also to create resistance so the movement stays really small.

Benefits: This is a great way to boost muscle tone in the cheeks, around the mouth and in the jaw to energize the skin. It also boosts circulation, which helps the cheeks to look brighter and healthier.

Weekly wellness hack Every time you are outside this week, look upward for an instant mood-booster. If it's daytime, look at the blue sky or clouds, and if it's night, look at the moon and stars. Make this a habit for this week – and for life. It puts everything into perspective and brings you calmly into the present moment.

My Positive Word for the Week:

....

The Way I Want to Feel this Week:

....

My Reason for Doing Face Yoga this Week:

....

"Find joy in the little things. Because these may just be the big things."

MONDAY

Today's intention:

....

When I did my Face Yoga today:

AM practice .... minutes   PM practice .... minutes

The areas I worked on today:

☐ Forehead ☐ Eyes ☐ Cheeks ☐ Mouth ☐ Jaw ☐ Neck ☐ Wellness

What I am most grateful for today:

....

....

TUESDAY

Today's intention:

....

When I did my Face Yoga today:

AM practice .... minutes   PM practice .... minutes

The areas I worked on today:

☐ Forehead ☐ Eyes ☐ Cheeks ☐ Mouth ☐ Jaw ☐ Neck ☐ Wellness

What I am most grateful for today:

....

....

WEDNESDAY

Today's intention:

....

When I did my Face Yoga today:

AM practice .... minutes   PM practice .... minutes

The areas I worked on today:

☐ Forehead ☐ Eyes ☐ Cheeks ☐ Mouth ☐ Jaw ☐ Neck ☐ Wellness

What I am most grateful for today:

....

....

THURSDAY

Today's intention:

....

When I did my Face Yoga today:

AM practice .... minutes   PM practice .... minutes

The areas I worked on today:

☐ Forehead ☐ Eyes ☐ Cheeks ☐ Mouth ☐ Jaw ☐ Neck ☐ Wellness

What I am most grateful for today:

....

....

FRIDAY

Today's intention:

....

When I did my Face Yoga today:

AM practice .... minutes   PM practice .... minutes

The areas I worked on today:

☐ Forehead ☐ Eyes ☐ Cheeks ☐ Mouth ☐ Jaw ☐ Neck ☐ Wellness

What I am most grateful for today:

....

....

SATURDAY

Today's intention:

....

When I did my Face Yoga today:

AM practice .... minutes   PM practice .... minutes

The areas I worked on today:

☐ Forehead ☐ Eyes ☐ Cheeks ☐ Mouth ☐ Jaw ☐ Neck ☐ Wellness

What I am most grateful for today:

....

....

SUNDAY

Today's intention:

....

When I did my Face Yoga today:

AM practice .... minutes   PM practice .... minutes

The areas I worked on today:

☐ Forehead ☐ Eyes ☐ Cheeks ☐ Mouth ☐ Jaw ☐ Neck ☐ Wellness

What I am most grateful for today:

....

....

What Went Well this Week:

....

....

What Didn't Go so Well this Week:

....

....

Week 18. Nurture

This week you will be focusing on the gentle nurturing qualities of your *chi* or *prana*. Your Face Yoga move is wonderful for helping the subtle energy to flow, which nurtures your skin, and your wellness hack uses scent to nurture deep within your soul.

TECHNIQUE OF THE WEEK
The Mouth Nurturing Technique

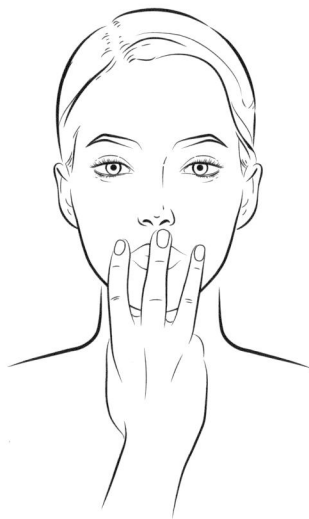

1. Using one hand, place your middle finger in your cupid's bow directly between the nose and mouth. Place your index and ring finger on the nasolabial folds. Hold for 30 seconds, breathing deeply, relaxing the whole face and feeling a sense of self-nurturing.

2. Then do a pulsing action, pressing your fingers down and then releasing at a rate of 1 per second for 20 rounds. Please note: the central acupressure point in the cupid's bow is a contraindication for pregnant women.

Benefits: This sequence helps to reduce tension around the mouth to prevent stress-related lines building up. It also stimulates acupressure points, which nurtures your wellbeing and helps to brighten tired or dull skin.

Weekly wellness hack Surround yourself with wonderful scents this week. It can be aromatherapy, seaside air, flowers, candles or even clean bedding or laundry. Indulge in the smell and allow it to help you feel nurtured as well as enhance your endorphins.

My Positive Word for the Week:

....

The Way I Want to Feel this Week:

....

My Reason for Doing Face Yoga this Week:

....

"Remember you need to nurture yourself just like you nurture others around you."

MONDAY

Today's intention:

....

When I did my Face Yoga today:

AM practice .... minutes   PM practice .... minutes

The areas I worked on today:

☐ Forehead ☐ Eyes ☐ Cheeks ☐ Mouth ☐ Jaw ☐ Neck ☐ Wellness

What I am most grateful for today:

....

....

TUESDAY

Today's intention:

....

When I did my Face Yoga today:

AM practice .... minutes   PM practice .... minutes

The areas I worked on today:

☐ Forehead ☐ Eyes ☐ Cheeks ☐ Mouth ☐ Jaw ☐ Neck ☐ Wellness

What I am most grateful for today:

....

....

WEDNESDAY

Today's intention:

....

When I did my Face Yoga today:

AM practice .... minutes   PM practice .... minutes

The areas I worked on today:

☐ Forehead ☐ Eyes ☐ Cheeks ☐ Mouth ☐ Jaw ☐ Neck ☐ Wellness

What I am most grateful for today:

....

....

THURSDAY

Today's intention:

....

When I did my Face Yoga today:

AM practice .... minutes   PM practice .... minutes

The areas I worked on today:

☐ Forehead ☐ Eyes ☐ Cheeks ☐ Mouth ☐ Jaw ☐ Neck ☐ Wellness

What I am most grateful for today:

....

....

FRIDAY

Today's intention:

....

When I did my Face Yoga today:

AM practice .... minutes   PM practice .... minutes

The areas I worked on today:

☐ Forehead ☐ Eyes ☐ Cheeks ☐ Mouth ☐ Jaw ☐ Neck ☐ Wellness

What I am most grateful for today:

....

....

SATURDAY

Today's intention:

....

When I did my Face Yoga today:

AM practice .... minutes   PM practice .... minutes

The areas I worked on today:

☐ Forehead ☐ Eyes ☐ Cheeks ☐ Mouth ☐ Jaw ☐ Neck ☐ Wellness

What I am most grateful for today:

....

....

SUNDAY

Today's intention:

....

When I did my Face Yoga today:

AM practice .... minutes   PM practice .... minutes

The areas I worked on today:

☐ Forehead ☐ Eyes ☐ Cheeks ☐ Mouth ☐ Jaw ☐ Neck ☐ Wellness

What I am most grateful for today:

....

....

What Went Well this Week:

....

....

What Didn't Go so Well this Week:

....

....

Week 19. Power

When we think of the word power, we often link it with control or domination. The true essence of power is about regaining your self-worth, your energy and truly living in your purpose. As you write your intentions this week, keep this thought in mind. Wearing white, using clear quartz and focusing on your crown chakra are great ways to step into the power of your intuition, your higher self and your true nature.

TECHNIQUE OF THE WEEK
The Jaw Powering Technique

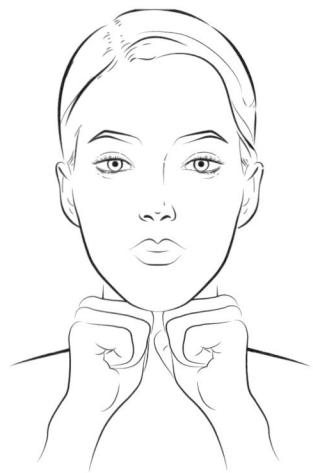

1. Bring your chin parallel to the floor and place both fists under your chin so the knuckles are touching. Keeping your lips closed, bring the tip of your tongue up toward the roof of your mouth at around a rate of 1 per second for 30 seconds. Create a feeling of your chin trying to move down but it can't due to your fists stopping it. Really feel the power of your jaw muscles against the resistance of your fists.

2. Rest for a few moments and then repeat a second time.

Benefits: This technique helps to tone the area under the chin through the powerful tongue movement, and the added resistance of the fists engages more of the jaw muscle to lift and firm.

> **Weekly wellness hack** Make a power playlist this week. Choose music that makes you feel strong, alive and empowered. Play it whenever you need to invoke these feelings.

My Positive Word for the Week:

....

The Way I Want to Feel this Week:

....

My Reason for Doing Face Yoga this Week:

....

"The strongest people rarely have an easy past."

MONDAY

Today's intention:

....

When I did my Face Yoga today:

AM practice .... minutes   PM practice .... minutes

The areas I worked on today:

☐ Forehead   ☐ Eyes   ☐ Cheeks   ☐ Mouth   ☐ Jaw   ☐ Neck   ☐ Wellness

What I am most grateful for today:

....

....

TUESDAY

Today's intention:

....

When I did my Face Yoga today:

AM practice .... minutes   PM practice .... minutes

The areas I worked on today:

☐ Forehead   ☐ Eyes   ☐ Cheeks   ☐ Mouth   ☐ Jaw   ☐ Neck   ☐ Wellness

What I am most grateful for today:

....

....

WEDNESDAY

Today's intention:

....

When I did my Face Yoga today:

AM practice .... minutes   PM practice .... minutes

The areas I worked on today:

☐ Forehead ☐ Eyes ☐ Cheeks ☐ Mouth ☐ Jaw ☐ Neck ☐ Wellness

What I am most grateful for today:

....

....

THURSDAY

Today's intention:

....

When I did my Face Yoga today:

AM practice .... minutes   PM practice .... minutes

The areas I worked on today:

☐ Forehead ☐ Eyes ☐ Cheeks ☐ Mouth ☐ Jaw ☐ Neck ☐ Wellness

What I am most grateful for today:

....

....

FRIDAY

Today's intention:

....

When I did my Face Yoga today:

AM practice .... minutes   PM practice .... minutes

The areas I worked on today:

☐ Forehead ☐ Eyes ☐ Cheeks ☐ Mouth ☐ Jaw ☐ Neck ☐ Wellness

What I am most grateful for today:

....

....

SATURDAY

Today's intention:

....

When I did my Face Yoga today:

AM practice .... minutes   PM practice .... minutes

The areas I worked on today:

☐ Forehead ☐ Eyes ☐ Cheeks ☐ Mouth ☐ Jaw ☐ Neck ☐ Wellness

What I am most grateful for today:

....

....

SUNDAY

Today's intention:

....

When I did my Face Yoga today:

AM practice .... minutes   PM practice .... minutes

The areas I worked on today:

☐ Forehead ☐ Eyes ☐ Cheeks ☐ Mouth ☐ Jaw ☐ Neck ☐ Wellness

What I am most grateful for today:

....

....

What Went Well this Week:

....

....

What Didn't Go so Well this Week:

....

....

Week 20. Comfort

Feeling comfortable in your own skin is a key element of The Danielle Collins Face Yoga Method. As you are now halfway through your second season, my hope is that all your hard work with your daily wellness and Face Yoga is helping you to feel this way. Your Face Yoga move this week brings physical comfort and your quote can bring emotional comfort to yourself and others.

TECHNIQUE OF THE WEEK
The Neck Comforting Technique

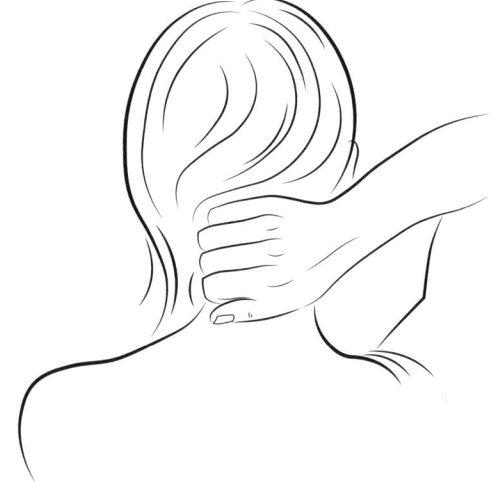

1. Grab hold of the back of your neck with one hand so your fingers are on one side of your spine and the heel of your hand is on the other. Squeeze the muscle as you slowly lift your hand away, really getting a deep release in the muscle.

2. Keep repeating this for 1 minute.

Benefits: This is a great way to reduce pain and tension in the back of the neck. As you regularly release these muscles, you will have less stress in your face and therefore fewer lines.

> **Weekly wellness hack** At night your skin and hair can get pulled and tugged around. Sleeping on a silk or satin pillowcase feels super comforting, plus it's a great way to wake up with a smoother face and hair.

My Positive Word for the Week:

....

The Way I Want to Feel this Week:

....

My Reason for Doing Face Yoga this Week:

....

"Kindness is key.
We all live under the same sky."

MONDAY

Today's intention:

....

When I did my Face Yoga today:

AM practice .... minutes   PM practice .... minutes

The areas I worked on today:

☐ Forehead   ☐ Eyes   ☐ Cheeks   ☐ Mouth   ☐ Jaw   ☐ Neck   ☐ Wellness

What I am most grateful for today:

....

....

TUESDAY

Today's intention:

....

When I did my Face Yoga today:

AM practice .... minutes   PM practice .... minutes

The areas I worked on today:

☐ Forehead   ☐ Eyes   ☐ Cheeks   ☐ Mouth   ☐ Jaw   ☐ Neck   ☐ Wellness

What I am most grateful for today:

....

....

WEDNESDAY

Today's intention:

....

When I did my Face Yoga today:

AM practice .... minutes   PM practice .... minutes

The areas I worked on today:

☐ Forehead ☐ Eyes ☐ Cheeks ☐ Mouth ☐ Jaw ☐ Neck ☐ Wellness

What I am most grateful for today:

....

....

THURSDAY

Today's intention:

....

When I did my Face Yoga today:

AM practice .... minutes   PM practice .... minutes

The areas I worked on today:

☐ Forehead ☐ Eyes ☐ Cheeks ☐ Mouth ☐ Jaw ☐ Neck ☐ Wellness

What I am most grateful for today:

....

....

FRIDAY

Today's intention:

....

When I did my Face Yoga today:

AM practice .... minutes   PM practice .... minutes

The areas I worked on today:

☐ Forehead ☐ Eyes ☐ Cheeks ☐ Mouth ☐ Jaw ☐ Neck ☐ Wellness

What I am most grateful for today:

....

....

SATURDAY

Today's intention:

....

When I did my Face Yoga today:

AM practice .... minutes   PM practice .... minutes

The areas I worked on today:

☐ Forehead ☐ Eyes ☐ Cheeks ☐ Mouth ☐ Jaw ☐ Neck ☐ Wellness

What I am most grateful for today:

....

....

SUNDAY

Today's intention:

....

When I did my Face Yoga today:

AM practice .... minutes   PM practice .... minutes

The areas I worked on today:

☐ Forehead ☐ Eyes ☐ Cheeks ☐ Mouth ☐ Jaw ☐ Neck ☐ Wellness

What I am most grateful for today:

....

....

What Went Well this Week:

....

....

What Didn't Go so Well this Week:

....

....

Week 21. Radiating

This week is about radiating energy to and from your skin, mind and body. Really connect to your sacral chakra and as you do your Face Yoga, visualize the vibrant colour of orange radiating from you. A study conducted in Japan in 2018 showed how facial exercise not only improved appearance but also improved mental health in participants. This week, focus on how Face Yoga can help radiate happiness, joy and energy.

TECHNIQUE OF THE WEEK
The Forehead Radiating Technique

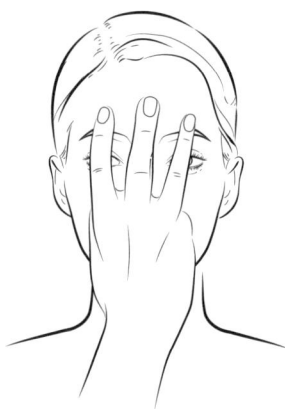

1. Using one hand, place your middle finger between your eyebrows, your index finger slightly above the middle of one eyebrow and your ring finger slightly above the middle of your other eyebrow. Gently wiggle your fingers on these points for 20 seconds.

2. Move your three fingers, still evenly spaced, to the middle of your forehead, wiggling them on these points for 20 seconds.

3. Move your three fingers to the top of your forehead by your hairline, wiggling them on these points for 20 seconds.

Benefits: These acupressure points can reduce stress, ease headaches and calm the mind. They are also wonderful for improving circulation, therefore helping collagen and elastin production, which in turn helps to smooth forehead lines and brighten the skin.

Weekly wellness hack Have fun with your Face Yoga this week and introduce a new facial tool to your routine, such as a gua sha, a crystal roller, a facial ice globe or a microcurrent device. Apply your serum and use your facial tool for 2 minutes after your Face Yoga for radiating skin.

My Positive Word for the Week:

....

The Way I Want to Feel this Week:

....

My Reason for Doing Face Yoga this Week:

....

"Something wonderful is about to happen to you. Always believe that."

MONDAY

Today's intention:

....

When I did my Face Yoga today:

AM practice .... minutes   PM practice .... minutes

The areas I worked on today:

☐ Forehead   ☐ Eyes   ☐ Cheeks   ☐ Mouth   ☐ Jaw   ☐ Neck   ☐ Wellness

What I am most grateful for today:

....

....

TUESDAY

Today's intention:

....

When I did my Face Yoga today:

AM practice .... minutes   PM practice .... minutes

The areas I worked on today:

☐ Forehead   ☐ Eyes   ☐ Cheeks   ☐ Mouth   ☐ Jaw   ☐ Neck   ☐ Wellness

What I am most grateful for today:

....

....

WEDNESDAY

Today's intention:

....

When I did my Face Yoga today:

AM practice .... minutes   PM practice .... minutes

The areas I worked on today:

☐ Forehead ☐ Eyes ☐ Cheeks ☐ Mouth ☐ Jaw ☐ Neck ☐ Wellness

What I am most grateful for today:

....

....

THURSDAY

Today's intention:

....

When I did my Face Yoga today:

AM practice .... minutes   PM practice .... minutes

The areas I worked on today:

☐ Forehead ☐ Eyes ☐ Cheeks ☐ Mouth ☐ Jaw ☐ Neck ☐ Wellness

What I am most grateful for today:

....

....

FRIDAY

Today's intention:

....

When I did my Face Yoga today:

AM practice .... minutes   PM practice .... minutes

The areas I worked on today:

☐ Forehead   ☐ Eyes   ☐ Cheeks   ☐ Mouth   ☐ Jaw   ☐ Neck   ☐ Wellness

What I am most grateful for today:

....

....

SATURDAY

Today's intention:

....

When I did my Face Yoga today:

AM practice .... minutes   PM practice .... minutes

The areas I worked on today:

☐ Forehead   ☐ Eyes   ☐ Cheeks   ☐ Mouth   ☐ Jaw   ☐ Neck   ☐ Wellness

What I am most grateful for today:

....

....

SUNDAY

Today's intention:

....

When I did my Face Yoga today:

AM practice .... minutes   PM practice .... minutes

The areas I worked on today:

☐ Forehead   ☐ Eyes   ☐ Cheeks   ☐ Mouth   ☐ Jaw   ☐ Neck   ☐ Wellness

What I am most grateful for today:

....

....

What Went Well this Week:

....

....

What Didn't Go so Well this Week:

....

....

Week 22. Revitalization

Are you ready to fully step into your energy this week and fully revitalize? If so, the first place to start is with your gentle yet effective Face Yoga technique. Your goal this week is to focus on one of the best ways to revitalize – sleep – as well as using this week's quote to revitalize your mindset. Place your sunstone crystal by your bed or on your desk and use it to help you feel energized.

TECHNIQUE OF THE WEEK
The Eye Revitalizing Technique

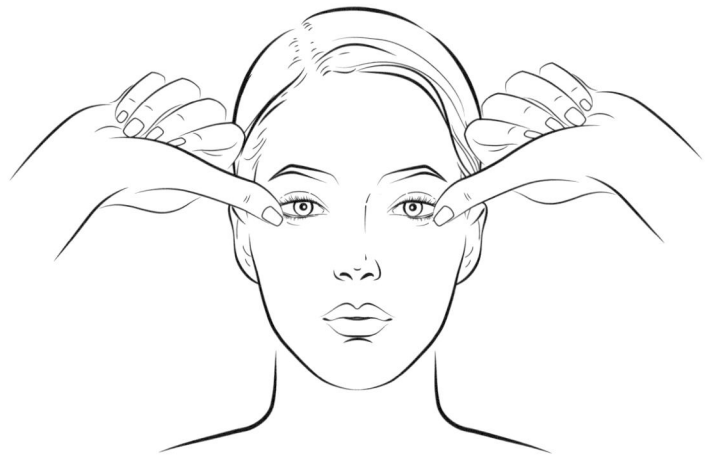

1. Using the pads of your thumbs, very lightly press the skin on the outer corners of your eyes and hold for 30 seconds.

2. Gently pulse your thumbs on these points for 30 seconds at a rate of 1 pulse per second (don't drag skin or press too hard).

Benefits: Using the thumbs on these points is often recommended in Ayurveda, as the thumbs project the main pranic energy of the hand. This means you can get deeper benefits, but you could use your index fingers if you prefer (which is how you will do many other acupressure points in this journal). Activating these points is a great way to revitalize tired, weak or stressed eyes. It also helps to ease tension and boost circulation in this area for revitalized and energized skin.

> **Weekly wellness hack** Turn off all technology at 7pm at least three evenings this week, and keep it off for at least 12 hours. This will help you sleep better and wake up revitalized. It gives your mind a chance to switch off from external stimulation and encourages you to spend your evenings doing other activities.

My Positive Word for the Week:

....

The Way I Want to Feel this Week:

....

My Reason for Doing Face Yoga this Week:

....

"Talk like you are blessed. Act like you are blessed. Feel like you are blessed. Then blessings will come."

MONDAY

Today's intention:

....

When I did my Face Yoga today:

AM practice .... minutes   PM practice .... minutes

The areas I worked on today:

☐ Forehead ☐ Eyes ☐ Cheeks ☐ Mouth ☐ Jaw ☐ Neck ☐ Wellness

What I am most grateful for today:

....

....

TUESDAY

Today's intention:

....

When I did my Face Yoga today:

AM practice .... minutes   PM practice .... minutes

The areas I worked on today:

☐ Forehead ☐ Eyes ☐ Cheeks ☐ Mouth ☐ Jaw ☐ Neck ☐ Wellness

What I am most grateful for today:

....

....

WEDNESDAY

Today's intention:

....

When I did my Face Yoga today:

AM practice .... minutes　　PM practice .... minutes

The areas I worked on today:

☐ Forehead ☐ Eyes ☐ Cheeks ☐ Mouth ☐ Jaw ☐ Neck ☐ Wellness

What I am most grateful for today:

....

....

THURSDAY

Today's intention:

....

When I did my Face Yoga today:

AM practice .... minutes　　PM practice .... minutes

The areas I worked on today:

☐ Forehead ☐ Eyes ☐ Cheeks ☐ Mouth ☐ Jaw ☐ Neck ☐ Wellness

What I am most grateful for today:

....

....

FRIDAY

Today's intention:

....

When I did my Face Yoga today:

AM practice .... minutes   PM practice .... minutes

The areas I worked on today:

☐ Forehead   ☐ Eyes   ☐ Cheeks   ☐ Mouth   ☐ Jaw   ☐ Neck   ☐ Wellness

What I am most grateful for today:

....

....

SATURDAY

Today's intention:

....

When I did my Face Yoga today:

AM practice .... minutes   PM practice .... minutes

The areas I worked on today:

☐ Forehead   ☐ Eyes   ☐ Cheeks   ☐ Mouth   ☐ Jaw   ☐ Neck   ☐ Wellness

What I am most grateful for today:

....

....

SUNDAY

Today's intention:

....

When I did my Face Yoga today:

AM practice .... minutes   PM practice .... minutes

The areas I worked on today:

☐ Forehead ☐ Eyes ☐ Cheeks ☐ Mouth ☐ Jaw ☐ Neck ☐ Wellness

What I am most grateful for today:

....

....

What Went Well this Week:

....

....

What Didn't Go so Well this Week:

....

....

Week 23. Glow

Glowing, energized skin is the goal of every Face Yoga technique in this journal. This week really aim to focus on this. If you aren't already in the habit, start taking weekly before and after photos to track your progress. This is also your week to really enjoy your skincare routine and use a mask to help your skin glow.

TECHNIQUE OF THE WEEK
The Cheek Glowing Technique

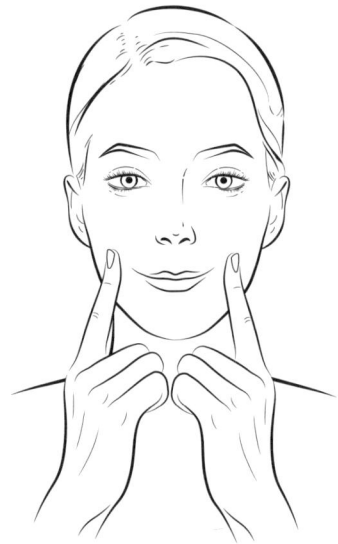

1. Slightly pull in your cheeks until you see and feel a little hollow in the centre. Place your index fingers in the indentation, then relax your cheeks completely. Hold for 30 seconds, applying medium pressure.

2. Make little circles with your index fingers in a clockwise direction for 15 seconds then in an anticlockwise direction for 15 seconds.

Benefits: Often referred to as the "glow point" this acupressure technique helps to promote better circulation for glowing cheeks. It also helps to ease tension from your cheeks and jaw for less pain, fewer stress-related wrinkles and a calmer mind. Researchers have found that facial massage on areas like this significantly improves blood circulation, blood flow and vascular function – all contributing to glowing skin.

Weekly wellness hack Pick a few days this week to take some time to use a face mask. The best time to do it is after cleansing (it can be a cream or sheet mask) and before your Face Yoga. Lie down and breathe for 10 minutes whilst the nourishing ingredients work their magic. Wash off then tone and moisturize.

My Positive Word for the Week:

....

The Way I Want to Feel this Week:

....

My Reason for Doing Face Yoga this Week:

....

"Don't dim your light any longer. It's your time to shine."

MONDAY

Today's intention:

....

When I did my Face Yoga today:

AM practice .... minutes   PM practice .... minutes

The areas I worked on today:

☐ Forehead ☐ Eyes ☐ Cheeks ☐ Mouth ☐ Jaw ☐ Neck ☐ Wellness

What I am most grateful for today:

....

....

TUESDAY

Today's intention:

....

When I did my Face Yoga today:

AM practice .... minutes   PM practice .... minutes

The areas I worked on today:

☐ Forehead ☐ Eyes ☐ Cheeks ☐ Mouth ☐ Jaw ☐ Neck ☐ Wellness

What I am most grateful for today:

....

....

WEDNESDAY

Today's intention:

....

When I did my Face Yoga today:

AM practice .... minutes   PM practice .... minutes

The areas I worked on today:

☐ Forehead ☐ Eyes ☐ Cheeks ☐ Mouth ☐ Jaw ☐ Neck ☐ Wellness

What I am most grateful for today:

....

....

THURSDAY

Today's intention:

....

When I did my Face Yoga today:

AM practice .... minutes   PM practice .... minutes

The areas I worked on today:

☐ Forehead ☐ Eyes ☐ Cheeks ☐ Mouth ☐ Jaw ☐ Neck ☐ Wellness

What I am most grateful for today:

....

....

FRIDAY

Today's intention:

....

When I did my Face Yoga today:

AM practice .... minutes   PM practice .... minutes

The areas I worked on today:

☐ Forehead ☐ Eyes ☐ Cheeks ☐ Mouth ☐ Jaw ☐ Neck ☐ Wellness

What I am most grateful for today:

....

....

SATURDAY

Today's intention:

....

When I did my Face Yoga today:

AM practice .... minutes   PM practice .... minutes

The areas I worked on today:

☐ Forehead ☐ Eyes ☐ Cheeks ☐ Mouth ☐ Jaw ☐ Neck ☐ Wellness

What I am most grateful for today:

....

....

SUNDAY

Today's intention:

....

When I did my Face Yoga today:

AM practice .... minutes   PM practice .... minutes

The areas I worked on today:

☐ Forehead   ☐ Eyes   ☐ Cheeks   ☐ Mouth   ☐ Jaw   ☐ Neck   ☐ Wellness

What I am most grateful for today:

....

....

What Went Well this Week:

....

....

What Didn't Go so Well this Week:

....

....

Week 24. Settling

Even just the thought of settling may make you sigh with relief. It's about letting go, coming to your stillness centre and letting your subtle energy flow through you. As you write your positive word and your goals for the week, make sure you feel fully settled first. Take some time to breathe deeply, perhaps snuggle in a blanket and have a warm drink. Then, when in a settled state, set your intentions, writing from your true inner voice.

TECHNIQUE OF THE WEEK
The Mouth Settling Technique

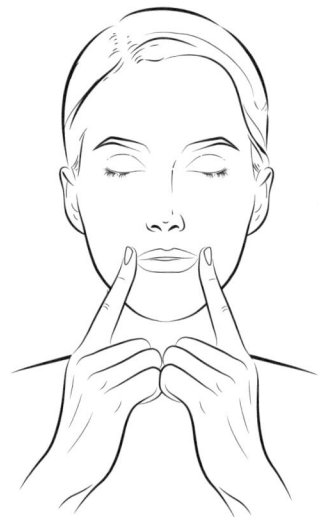

1. Using both hands, place your index fingers on the corners of your mouth, making sure your face is in a neutral and settled state. Hold here for 30 seconds and breathe deeply.

2. Massage in a small circular clockwise motion for 15 seconds and anticlockwise motion for another 15 seconds.

Benefits: In facial reflexology this point is said to be related to the lung area. It can settle, balance and nourish, and it's also great for helping soften lines by encouraging circulation as well as *prana* or energy/life force to this area.

> **Weekly wellness hack** Set an alarm on your phone for every three hours during the day, and when it goes off take a moment to soften your jaw, unfurrow your brow, relax your shoulders and lengthen your neck. Get to know this settled position and come back to it often.

My Positive Word for the Week:

....

The Way I Want to Feel this Week:

....

My Reason for Doing Face Yoga this Week:

....

"We are human beings. Not human doings."

MONDAY

Today's intention:

....

When I did my Face Yoga today:

AM practice .... minutes   PM practice .... minutes

The areas I worked on today:

☐ Forehead ☐ Eyes ☐ Cheeks ☐ Mouth ☐ Jaw ☐ Neck ☐ Wellness

What I am most grateful for today:

....

....

TUESDAY

Today's intention:

....

When I did my Face Yoga today:

AM practice .... minutes   PM practice .... minutes

The areas I worked on today:

☐ Forehead ☐ Eyes ☐ Cheeks ☐ Mouth ☐ Jaw ☐ Neck ☐ Wellness

What I am most grateful for today:

....

....

WEDNESDAY

Today's intention:

....

When I did my Face Yoga today:

AM practice .... minutes   PM practice .... minutes

The areas I worked on today:

☐ Forehead ☐ Eyes ☐ Cheeks ☐ Mouth ☐ Jaw ☐ Neck ☐ Wellness

What I am most grateful for today:

....

....

THURSDAY

Today's intention:

....

When I did my Face Yoga today:

AM practice .... minutes   PM practice .... minutes

The areas I worked on today:

☐ Forehead ☐ Eyes ☐ Cheeks ☐ Mouth ☐ Jaw ☐ Neck ☐ Wellness

What I am most grateful for today:

....

....

FRIDAY

Today's intention:

....

When I did my Face Yoga today:

AM practice .... minutes   PM practice .... minutes

The areas I worked on today:

☐ Forehead ☐ Eyes ☐ Cheeks ☐ Mouth ☐ Jaw ☐ Neck ☐ Wellness

What I am most grateful for today:

....

....

SATURDAY

Today's intention:

....

When I did my Face Yoga today:

AM practice .... minutes   PM practice .... minutes

The areas I worked on today:

☐ Forehead ☐ Eyes ☐ Cheeks ☐ Mouth ☐ Jaw ☐ Neck ☐ Wellness

What I am most grateful for today:

....

....

SUNDAY

Today's intention:

....

When I did my Face Yoga today:

AM practice .... minutes   PM practice .... minutes

The areas I worked on today:

☐ Forehead ☐ Eyes ☐ Cheeks ☐ Mouth ☐ Jaw ☐ Neck ☐ Wellness

What I am most grateful for today:

....

....

What Went Well this Week:

....

....

What Didn't Go so Well this Week:

....

....

Week 25. Release

Releasing stress from the mind, body and face is imperative to looking and feeling youthful. The sacral chakra, located about 7.5cm/3in below the naval, is your emotional centre, so this week start by tuning in to this area and ask yourself the question: "What do I need to release this week?" Really listen to the answer. Your Face Yoga is an incredible way of releasing the stress that manifests itself in the jaw area, often when we are emotionally holding on too tight.

TECHNIQUE OF THE WEEK
The Jaw Releasing Technique

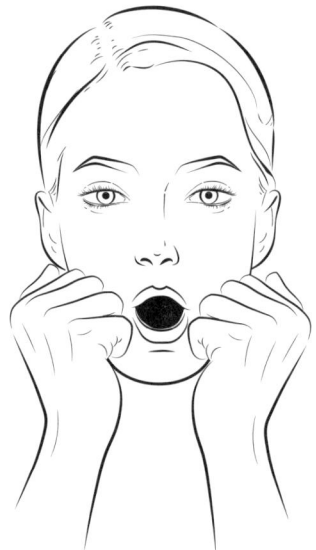

1. Make both hands into fists and place your finger joints under the highest part of your cheekbones so the index finger joint is closest to your ears. Start to open and close your mouth slowly, using a mirror to check alignment.

2. Continue for 1 minute.

Benefits: As you do this, you should feel a lot of tension come to the surface and then dissipate. It shouldn't feel painful but if you have a very tight jaw or TMJ disorder, it may feel intense so ease off if you need to. This technique is great for releasing pain and tightness in the jaw area, which also reduces tension-induced lines. Additionally, it helps to tone the area around the mouth and the massage is great for boosting circulation for brighter skin.

> **Weekly wellness hack** Spend some time this week doing an audit of your social media (if you use it): unfollow any account that isn't inspiring or informative and doesn't invoke joy, and then start to follow accounts that make you feel good. You'll feel a release of negativity.

My Positive Word for the Week:

....

The Way I Want to Feel this Week:

....

My Reason for Doing Face Yoga this Week:

....

"If you feel like everyone has a perfect plan or knows exactly what they are doing, release that thought – they are probably struggling too and thinking the same thing."

MONDAY

Today's intention:

....

When I did my Face Yoga today:

AM practice .... minutes   PM practice .... minutes

The areas I worked on today:

☐ Forehead   ☐ Eyes   ☐ Cheeks   ☐ Mouth   ☐ Jaw   ☐ Neck   ☐ Wellness

What I am most grateful for today:

....

....

TUESDAY

Today's intention:

....

When I did my Face Yoga today:

AM practice .... minutes   PM practice .... minutes

The areas I worked on today:

☐ Forehead   ☐ Eyes   ☐ Cheeks   ☐ Mouth   ☐ Jaw   ☐ Neck   ☐ Wellness

What I am most grateful for today:

....

....

WEDNESDAY

Today's intention:

....

When I did my Face Yoga today:

AM practice .... minutes   PM practice .... minutes

The areas I worked on today:

☐ Forehead ☐ Eyes ☐ Cheeks ☐ Mouth ☐ Jaw ☐ Neck ☐ Wellness

What I am most grateful for today:

....

....

THURSDAY

Today's intention:

....

When I did my Face Yoga today:

AM practice .... minutes   PM practice .... minutes

The areas I worked on today:

☐ Forehead ☐ Eyes ☐ Cheeks ☐ Mouth ☐ Jaw ☐ Neck ☐ Wellness

What I am most grateful for today:

....

....

FRIDAY

Today's intention:

....

When I did my Face Yoga today:

AM practice .... minutes   PM practice .... minutes

The areas I worked on today:

☐ Forehead ☐ Eyes ☐ Cheeks ☐ Mouth ☐ Jaw ☐ Neck ☐ Wellness

What I am most grateful for today:

....

....

SATURDAY

Today's intention:

....

When I did my Face Yoga today:

AM practice .... minutes   PM practice .... minutes

The areas I worked on today:

☐ Forehead ☐ Eyes ☐ Cheeks ☐ Mouth ☐ Jaw ☐ Neck ☐ Wellness

What I am most grateful for today:

....

....

SUNDAY

Today's intention:

....

When I did my Face Yoga today:

AM practice .... minutes   PM practice .... minutes

The areas I worked on today:

☐ Forehead ☐ Eyes ☐ Cheeks ☐ Mouth ☐ Jaw ☐ Neck ☐ Wellness

What I am most grateful for today:

....

....

What Went Well this Week:

....

....

What Didn't Go so Well this Week:

....

....

Week 26. Activation

Congratulations, you are nearly halfway through your year! You have done 25 weeks of Face Yoga and wellness. The final week of this season is about activating the upper body and lower face to tone, release and energize. Use your deep breathing and bring your clear quartz crystal into your space, as this will help balance the crown chakra which is linked to presence, connection, consciousness and wisdom.

TECHNIQUE OF THE WEEK
The Neck Activating Technique

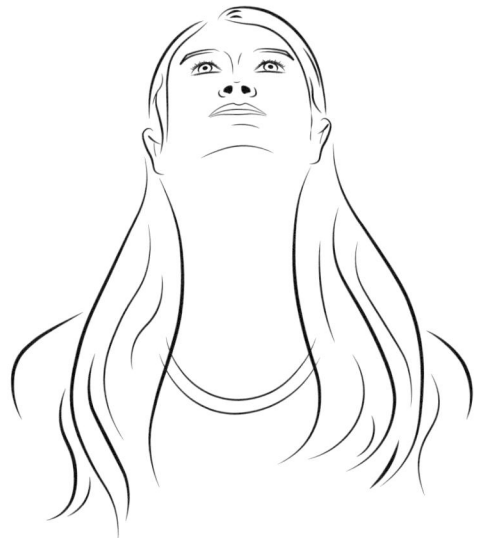

1. Clasp your hands behind your back, squeeze your shoulder blades together and open your chest. Gently tilt your head back as far as is comfortable. Bring your tongue up to the roof of your mouth, then relax it back down. Repeat 30 times.

2. Relax and repeat the sequence again.

Benefits: This helps to firm loose skin under the chin, tone the neck and release shoulder tension. It opens and activates tight and lesser-used chest muscles in the upper body.

> **Weekly wellness hack** This week try one new type of exercise or activity that you haven't tried before or haven't done for a while. Notice how it activates and remotivates your mind, wakes up your body and brings you a sense of fun and joy.

My Positive Word for the Week:

....

The Way I Want to Feel this Week:

....

My Reason for Doing Face Yoga this Week:

....

"Don't measure your progress using someone else's ruler."

MONDAY

Today's intention:

....

When I did my Face Yoga today:

AM practice .... minutes   PM practice .... minutes

The areas I worked on today:

☐ Forehead   ☐ Eyes   ☐ Cheeks   ☐ Mouth   ☐ Jaw   ☐ Neck   ☐ Wellness

What I am most grateful for today:

....

....

TUESDAY

Today's intention:

....

When I did my Face Yoga today:

AM practice .... minutes   PM practice .... minutes

The areas I worked on today:

☐ Forehead   ☐ Eyes   ☐ Cheeks   ☐ Mouth   ☐ Jaw   ☐ Neck   ☐ Wellness

What I am most grateful for today:

....

....

WEDNESDAY

Today's intention:

....

When I did my Face Yoga today:

AM practice .... minutes   PM practice .... minutes

The areas I worked on today:

☐ Forehead ☐ Eyes ☐ Cheeks ☐ Mouth ☐ Jaw ☐ Neck ☐ Wellness

What I am most grateful for today:

....

....

THURSDAY

Today's intention:

....

When I did my Face Yoga today:

AM practice .... minutes   PM practice .... minutes

The areas I worked on today:

☐ Forehead ☐ Eyes ☐ Cheeks ☐ Mouth ☐ Jaw ☐ Neck ☐ Wellness

What I am most grateful for today:

....

....

FRIDAY

Today's intention:

....

When I did my Face Yoga today:

AM practice .... minutes   PM practice .... minutes

The areas I worked on today:

☐ Forehead ☐ Eyes ☐ Cheeks ☐ Mouth ☐ Jaw ☐ Neck ☐ Wellness

What I am most grateful for today:

....

....

SATURDAY

Today's intention:

....

When I did my Face Yoga today:

AM practice .... minutes   PM practice .... minutes

The areas I worked on today:

☐ Forehead ☐ Eyes ☐ Cheeks ☐ Mouth ☐ Jaw ☐ Neck ☐ Wellness

What I am most grateful for today:

....

....

SUNDAY

Today's intention:

....

When I did my Face Yoga today:

AM practice .... minutes   PM practice .... minutes

The areas I worked on today:

☐ Forehead ☐ Eyes ☐ Cheeks ☐ Mouth ☐ Jaw ☐ Neck ☐ Wellness

What I am most grateful for today:

....

....

What Went Well this Week:

....

....

What Didn't Go so Well this Week:

....

....

Season 3
Lift your face

Happiness chemical: dopamine
Chakra: third eye chakra
Crystal: amethyst
Colour: indigo

Mantra: "I see, trust and know my own inner and outer beauty."

If I had to pick one key aesthetic benefit of Face Yoga, it would be that it lifts the skin. A significant part of Face Yoga is focused on toning, strengthening and lifting the muscles in the face and therefore lifting the skin attached. As we age we naturally lose muscle tone as well as collagen and elastin, which can mean the skin can look less lifted. Face Yoga works on strengthening muscle and boosting collagen and elastin production. A 2018 study by Northwestern University showed that 30 minutes of Face Yoga per day for 20 weeks made participants look 3 years younger. What was most notable was the lifting benefits for the lower face.

Over the next 13 weeks you will also be focusing on lifting your mood and spirit to feel great. Dopamine is released when we do things which uplift us and give us pleasure. It is known as the reward chemical as it is often released when we are satisfied with what we have done. As you tick your boxes for the areas of the face that you have worked on, notice how it lifts your spirit and feels good – that's your dopamine!

This season is focused on just one chakra: the third eye. This is the only chakra located on the face, so it's a very significant one in Face Yoga. It's all about intuition. Intuition is an important part of Face Yoga and wellness as a whole. As you tap into your intuition, you will find the answers to questions such as, "What does my face need?", "How is my mind truly feeling?" and "What is my body trying to tell me?" Take a few moments to breathe, maybe whilst holding an amethyst or wearing the colour indigo, and ask yourself these questions. Let the answers guide your daily journalling this season, as well as guide you through your lifting Face Yoga routines.

All the weekly themes help to lift your face. True lifting encompasses so many aspects, which you will work on each week over the next 13 weeks.

Week 27. Opening

Before we lift we must open. This week is about opening your face to relieve tension and stress, giving space and air to your skin and opening your heart and mind. One way to open your mind is by using your seasonal mantra each day this week to set the tone for the rest of the season.

TECHNIQUE OF THE WEEK
The Face Opening Technique

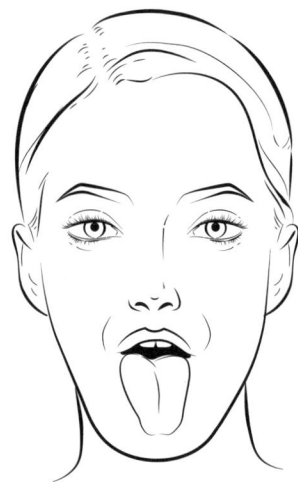

1. Bring your hands up to your face and make them into fists. Close your eyes, inhale through your nose and slightly tense the face without crumpling it up or causing lines.

2. Exhale deeply and as you do, open your mouth, stick out your tongue as much as possible, open your eyes, open your chest, open your hands wide and slightly look up with your eyes.

3. Continue this breath sequence for 1 minute, extending the exhale each time.

Benefits: This classic Face Yoga move, often called "the lion", helps your face to look and feel healthy, tension-free and open. It is great to do if you feel stressed or if your face is looking dull or tired.

> **Weekly wellness hack** This week pick two days to go makeup free. Wear SPF but nothing else. This will not only allow your skin to have a break from an overload of products but it will open your mind and heart to not wearing a mask.

My Positive Word for the Week:

....

The Way I Want to Feel this Week:

....

My Reason for Doing Face Yoga this Week:

....

"Open your heart, open your mind. You never know what you may find."

MONDAY

Today's intention:

....

When I did my Face Yoga today:

AM practice .... minutes   PM practice .... minutes

The areas I worked on today:

☐ Forehead ☐ Eyes ☐ Cheeks ☐ Mouth ☐ Jaw ☐ Neck ☐ Wellness

What I am most grateful for today:

....

....

TUESDAY

Today's intention:

....

When I did my Face Yoga today:

AM practice .... minutes   PM practice .... minutes

The areas I worked on today:

☐ Forehead ☐ Eyes ☐ Cheeks ☐ Mouth ☐ Jaw ☐ Neck ☐ Wellness

What I am most grateful for today:

....

....

WEDNESDAY

Today's intention:

....

When I did my Face Yoga today:

AM practice .... minutes   PM practice .... minutes

The areas I worked on today:

☐ Forehead ☐ Eyes ☐ Cheeks ☐ Mouth ☐ Jaw ☐ Neck ☐ Wellness

What I am most grateful for today:

....

....

THURSDAY

Today's intention:

....

When I did my Face Yoga today:

AM practice .... minutes   PM practice .... minutes

The areas I worked on today:

☐ Forehead ☐ Eyes ☐ Cheeks ☐ Mouth ☐ Jaw ☐ Neck ☐ Wellness

What I am most grateful for today:

....

....

FRIDAY

Today's intention:

....

When I did my Face Yoga today:

AM practice .... minutes   PM practice .... minutes

The areas I worked on today:

☐ Forehead ☐ Eyes ☐ Cheeks ☐ Mouth ☐ Jaw ☐ Neck ☐ Wellness

What I am most grateful for today:

....

....

SATURDAY

Today's intention:

....

When I did my Face Yoga today:

AM practice .... minutes   PM practice .... minutes

The areas I worked on today:

☐ Forehead ☐ Eyes ☐ Cheeks ☐ Mouth ☐ Jaw ☐ Neck ☐ Wellness

What I am most grateful for today:

....

....

SUNDAY

Today's intention:

....

When I did my Face Yoga today:

AM practice .... minutes   PM practice .... minutes

The areas I worked on today:

☐ Forehead   ☐ Eyes   ☐ Cheeks   ☐ Mouth   ☐ Jaw   ☐ Neck   ☐ Wellness

What I am most grateful for today:

....

....

What Went Well this Week:

....

....

What Didn't Go so Well this Week:

....

....

Week 28. Sculpting

One of the key benefits of Face Yoga is that it helps sculpt the face to enhance features and add definition. This week's Face Yoga is designed to sculpt and lift the eyebrows and the forehead, and this week's wellness hack is about sculpting the body through yoga.

TECHNIQUE OF THE WEEK
The Forehead Sculpting Technique

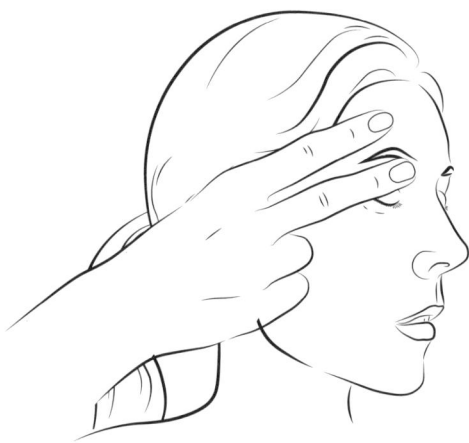

1. Using one hand, place your middle and index fingers on your third eye point between the eyebrows (so your fingers are horizontal) and smooth them outward along one of your eyebrows to your temple. Your index finger should be moving along the top of your eyebrow and your middle finger should be moving just under the eyebrow. Slightly squeeze your eyebrow as you move but be careful not to drag the delicate skin. When you reach the temple, lift off.

2. Repeat this sculpting massage for 30 seconds.

3. Repeat on the other side for 30 seconds.

Benefits: This helps your forehead to look more sculpted as it lifts, shapes and firms your eyebrows. It is also great for easing strain and tension from your eyebrow area.

> **Weekly wellness hack** This week, incorporate yoga into your routine to help sculpt your body. You may already be a regular yogi and if so, for the next seven days, focus on your favourite strengthening poses which help you sculpt your muscles.

My Positive Word for the Week:

....

The Way I Want to Feel this Week:

....

My Reason for Doing Face Yoga this Week:

....

"Self-care isn't selfish. Self-love isn't selfish. Self-appreciation isn't selfish."

MONDAY

Today's intention:

....

When I did my Face Yoga today:

AM practice .... minutes   PM practice .... minutes

The areas I worked on today:

☐ Forehead   ☐ Eyes   ☐ Cheeks   ☐ Mouth   ☐ Jaw   ☐ Neck   ☐ Wellness

What I am most grateful for today:

....

....

TUESDAY

Today's intention:

....

When I did my Face Yoga today:

AM practice .... minutes   PM practice .... minutes

The areas I worked on today:

☐ Forehead   ☐ Eyes   ☐ Cheeks   ☐ Mouth   ☐ Jaw   ☐ Neck   ☐ Wellness

What I am most grateful for today:

....

....

WEDNESDAY

Today's intention:

....

When I did my Face Yoga today:

AM practice .... minutes   PM practice .... minutes

The areas I worked on today:

☐ Forehead   ☐ Eyes   ☐ Cheeks   ☐ Mouth   ☐ Jaw   ☐ Neck   ☐ Wellness

What I am most grateful for today:

....

....

THURSDAY

Today's intention:

....

When I did my Face Yoga today:

AM practice .... minutes   PM practice .... minutes

The areas I worked on today:

☐ Forehead   ☐ Eyes   ☐ Cheeks   ☐ Mouth   ☐ Jaw   ☐ Neck   ☐ Wellness

What I am most grateful for today:

....

....

FRIDAY

Today's intention:

....

When I did my Face Yoga today:

AM practice .... minutes   PM practice .... minutes

The areas I worked on today:

☐ Forehead ☐ Eyes ☐ Cheeks ☐ Mouth ☐ Jaw ☐ Neck ☐ Wellness

What I am most grateful for today:

....

....

SATURDAY

Today's intention:

....

When I did my Face Yoga today:

AM practice .... minutes   PM practice .... minutes

The areas I worked on today:

☐ Forehead ☐ Eyes ☐ Cheeks ☐ Mouth ☐ Jaw ☐ Neck ☐ Wellness

What I am most grateful for today:

....

....

SUNDAY

Today's intention:

....

When I did my Face Yoga today:

AM practice .... minutes   PM practice .... minutes

The areas I worked on today:

☐ Forehead ☐ Eyes ☐ Cheeks ☐ Mouth ☐ Jaw ☐ Neck ☐ Wellness

What I am most grateful for today:

....

....

What Went Well this Week:

....

....

What Didn't Go so Well this Week:

....

....

Week 29. Firming

This week is all about firming. By now, you might have a good daily routine of many Face Yoga moves, most of which help to firm, so this week's technique is great to add to your repertoire. As well as firming, you are affirming exactly what your face and body need. This wellness hack allows you to balance your third eye chakra to access your intuition, so as you do this, wear indigo or hold your amethyst.

TECHNIQUE OF THE WEEK
The Eye Firming Technique

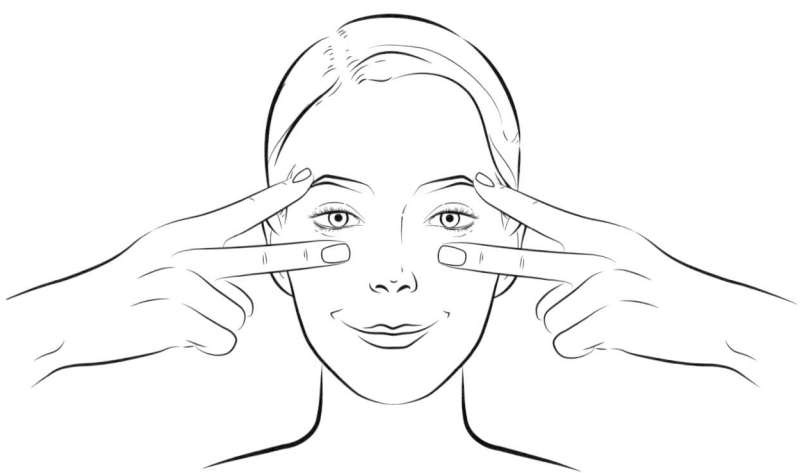

1. Using both hands, place your index fingers in a horizontal position on the outer edge of your eyebrows, slightly smoothing the skin, and place your middle fingers, also horizontally, just under your eyes on the bone. Making sure no lines are created on your forehead or around your eyes, half close your eyes, aiming to feel a little shake or pulse. Hold for 2 seconds, and then open your eyes.

2. Keep repeating this exercise for 1 minute.

Benefits: This technique, when done regularly, helps to firm the orbicularis oculi muscle around the eye. This can lift the eye area, preventing and reducing lines and wrinkles under the eye and around the outer edges of the eye.

> **Weekly wellness hack** With this week's wellness hack, you are affirming exactly what your face and body need. Simply close your eyes, focus on your third eye point, then ask yourself, "What does my face and body need in this moment?" and listen to the answer. You will learn a lot!

My Positive Word for the Week:

....

The Way I Want to Feel this Week:

....

My Reason for Doing Face Yoga this Week:

....

"*Change is scary. It's unknown. It's uncomfortable. But sometimes we need change and we must find the courage to do it.*"

MONDAY

Today's intention:

....

When I did my Face Yoga today:

AM practice .... minutes   PM practice .... minutes

The areas I worked on today:

☐ Forehead ☐ Eyes ☐ Cheeks ☐ Mouth ☐ Jaw ☐ Neck ☐ Wellness

What I am most grateful for today:

....

....

TUESDAY

Today's intention:

....

When I did my Face Yoga today:

AM practice .... minutes   PM practice .... minutes

The areas I worked on today:

☐ Forehead ☐ Eyes ☐ Cheeks ☐ Mouth ☐ Jaw ☐ Neck ☐ Wellness

What I am most grateful for today:

....

....

WEDNESDAY

Today's intention:

....

When I did my Face Yoga today:

AM practice .... minutes   PM practice .... minutes

The areas I worked on today:

☐ Forehead   ☐ Eyes   ☐ Cheeks   ☐ Mouth   ☐ Jaw   ☐ Neck   ☐ Wellness

What I am most grateful for today:

....

....

THURSDAY

Today's intention:

....

When I did my Face Yoga today:

AM practice .... minutes   PM practice .... minutes

The areas I worked on today:

☐ Forehead   ☐ Eyes   ☐ Cheeks   ☐ Mouth   ☐ Jaw   ☐ Neck   ☐ Wellness

What I am most grateful for today:

....

....

FRIDAY

Today's intention:

....

When I did my Face Yoga today:

AM practice .... minutes   PM practice .... minutes

The areas I worked on today:

☐ Forehead   ☐ Eyes   ☐ Cheeks   ☐ Mouth   ☐ Jaw   ☐ Neck   ☐ Wellness

What I am most grateful for today:

....

....

SATURDAY

Today's intention:

....

When I did my Face Yoga today:

AM practice .... minutes   PM practice .... minutes

The areas I worked on today:

☐ Forehead   ☐ Eyes   ☐ Cheeks   ☐ Mouth   ☐ Jaw   ☐ Neck   ☐ Wellness

What I am most grateful for today:

....

....

SUNDAY

Today's intention:

....

When I did my Face Yoga today:

AM practice .... minutes   PM practice .... minutes

The areas I worked on today:

☐ Forehead ☐ Eyes ☐ Cheeks ☐ Mouth ☐ Jaw ☐ Neck ☐ Wellness

What I am most grateful for today:

....

....

What Went Well this Week:

....

....

What Didn't Go so Well this Week:

....

....

Week 30. Freshening

The massage aspect of Face Yoga is a highly effective way to help the skin look and feel lifted and fresher. A 2016 study on facial massage showed that it "revealed marked morphological changes of the nasolabial folds". This week, this is the exact area you will be massaging (and freshening). Remember, fresh skin also comes from what we eat, so this is what this week's wellness hack will focus on.

TECHNIQUE OF THE WEEK
The Cheek Freshening Technique

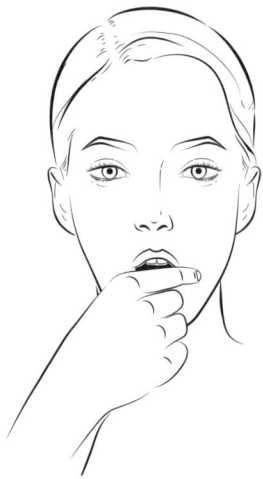

1. Starting with super-clean hands, place the thumb of one hand inside the opposite corner of your mouth and place your index finger on the outside of your mouth just below the corner (where smile lines often start). Using both fingers together, one inside the mouth and one outside, smooth upward and lift off near the top of your nasolabial fold.

2. Go back to your starting position and repeat for 30 seconds

3. Swap hands and repeat on the other side for 30 seconds.

Benefits: Working inside your mouth is a powerful way to lift and firm muscle, smooth lines and ease tension. Your skin will look brighter and fresher and nasolabial folds will be less visible with regular practice.

> **Weekly wellness hack** Freshen up your healthy habits (and your skin) by trying a new fruit or vegetable. It can be one you have never tried before or one you rarely eat. This can be beneficial for your gut microbiome and your nutrient levels, and trying something new can spark creativity when it comes to your meals and snacks.

My Positive Word for the Week:

....

The Way I Want to Feel this Week:

....

My Reason for Doing Face Yoga this Week:

....

"Happy skin starts with happiness within."

MONDAY

Today's intention:

....

When I did my Face Yoga today:

AM practice .... minutes   PM practice .... minutes

The areas I worked on today:

☐ Forehead   ☐ Eyes   ☐ Cheeks   ☐ Mouth   ☐ Jaw   ☐ Neck   ☐ Wellness

What I am most grateful for today:

....

....

TUESDAY

Today's intention:

....

When I did my Face Yoga today:

AM practice .... minutes   PM practice .... minutes

The areas I worked on today:

☐ Forehead   ☐ Eyes   ☐ Cheeks   ☐ Mouth   ☐ Jaw   ☐ Neck   ☐ Wellness

What I am most grateful for today:

....

....

WEDNESDAY

Today's intention:

....

When I did my Face Yoga today:

AM practice .... minutes   PM practice .... minutes

The areas I worked on today:

☐ Forehead   ☐ Eyes   ☐ Cheeks   ☐ Mouth   ☐ Jaw   ☐ Neck   ☐ Wellness

What I am most grateful for today:

....

....

THURSDAY

Today's intention:

....

When I did my Face Yoga today:

AM practice .... minutes   PM practice .... minutes

The areas I worked on today:

☐ Forehead   ☐ Eyes   ☐ Cheeks   ☐ Mouth   ☐ Jaw   ☐ Neck   ☐ Wellness

What I am most grateful for today:

....

....

FRIDAY

Today's intention:

....

When I did my Face Yoga today:

AM practice .... minutes   PM practice .... minutes

The areas I worked on today:

☐ Forehead ☐ Eyes ☐ Cheeks ☐ Mouth ☐ Jaw ☐ Neck ☐ Wellness

What I am most grateful for today:

....

....

SATURDAY

Today's intention:

....

When I did my Face Yoga today:

AM practice .... minutes   PM practice .... minutes

The areas I worked on today:

☐ Forehead ☐ Eyes ☐ Cheeks ☐ Mouth ☐ Jaw ☐ Neck ☐ Wellness

What I am most grateful for today:

....

....

SUNDAY

Today's intention:

....

When I did my Face Yoga today:

AM practice .... minutes   PM practice .... minutes

The areas I worked on today:

☐ Forehead ☐ Eyes ☐ Cheeks ☐ Mouth ☐ Jaw ☐ Neck ☐ Wellness

What I am most grateful for today:

....

....

What Went Well this Week:

....

....

What Didn't Go so Well this Week:

....

....

Week 31. Invigoration

When you invigorate your face from the inside out, as you will be doing with this week's Face Yoga technique, you will have healthier and more lifted skin. Your mind will also feel invigorated. Use your seasonal mantra as much as you can this week to further help you feel invigorated at a deep subconscious level.

The Mouth Invigorating Technique

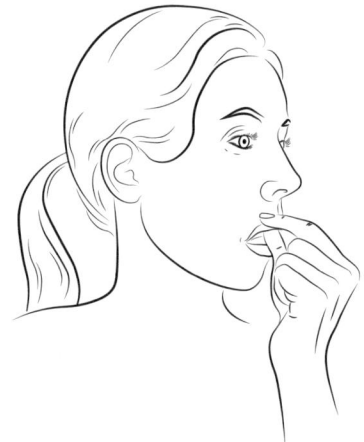

1. Starting with super-clean hands, place the index finger of one hand inside the corner of your mouth, just inside your lower lip. Place your thumb on the same place but on the outside. Gently squeeze your lip, then lift off. Move slightly along your bottom lip and do the same, then continue until you reach the opposite corner of your mouth.

2. Repeat in the other direction so you end up at your starting position.

3. Now move to your top lip, this time placing your thumb inside your top lip and your index finger on the outside, starting at the corner. Squeeze all along the top lip then back in the other direction.

Benefits: This works by invigorating and firing up your orbicularis oris muscle, which is great for circulation and healthy cell renewal. It is also wonderful for lifting the skin around your mouth.

> **Weekly wellness hack** This week is all about reinvigorating your love for yourself and finding ways to embrace your personality with all its quirks! As you go through the week, notice (and write down) what makes you so unique, what stands out about your personality and why others love you. It will really lift your spirits.

My Positive Word for the Week:

....

The Way I Want to Feel this Week:

....

My Reason for Doing Face Yoga this Week:

....

"So many people love you. Don't worry about those who don't."

MONDAY

Today's intention:

....

When I did my Face Yoga today:

AM practice .... minutes   PM practice .... minutes

The areas I worked on today:

☐ Forehead   ☐ Eyes   ☐ Cheeks   ☐ Mouth   ☐ Jaw   ☐ Neck   ☐ Wellness

What I am most grateful for today:

....

....

TUESDAY

Today's intention:

....

When I did my Face Yoga today:

AM practice .... minutes   PM practice .... minutes

The areas I worked on today:

☐ Forehead   ☐ Eyes   ☐ Cheeks   ☐ Mouth   ☐ Jaw   ☐ Neck   ☐ Wellness

What I am most grateful for today:

....

....

WEDNESDAY

Today's intention:

....

When I did my Face Yoga today:

AM practice .... minutes   PM practice .... minutes

The areas I worked on today:

☐ Forehead   ☐ Eyes   ☐ Cheeks   ☐ Mouth   ☐ Jaw   ☐ Neck   ☐ Wellness

What I am most grateful for today:

....

....

THURSDAY

Today's intention:

....

When I did my Face Yoga today:

AM practice .... minutes   PM practice .... minutes

The areas I worked on today:

☐ Forehead   ☐ Eyes   ☐ Cheeks   ☐ Mouth   ☐ Jaw   ☐ Neck   ☐ Wellness

What I am most grateful for today:

....

....

FRIDAY

Today's intention:

....

When I did my Face Yoga today:

AM practice .... minutes   PM practice .... minutes

The areas I worked on today:

☐ Forehead ☐ Eyes ☐ Cheeks ☐ Mouth ☐ Jaw ☐ Neck ☐ Wellness

What I am most grateful for today:

....

....

SATURDAY

Today's intention:

....

When I did my Face Yoga today:

AM practice .... minutes   PM practice .... minutes

The areas I worked on today:

☐ Forehead ☐ Eyes ☐ Cheeks ☐ Mouth ☐ Jaw ☐ Neck ☐ Wellness

What I am most grateful for today:

....

....

SUNDAY

Today's intention:

....

When I did my Face Yoga today:

AM practice .... minutes   PM practice .... minutes

The areas I worked on today:

☐ Forehead ☐ Eyes ☐ Cheeks ☐ Mouth ☐ Jaw ☐ Neck ☐ Wellness

What I am most grateful for today:

....

....

What Went Well this Week:

....

....

What Didn't Go so Well this Week:

....

....

Week 32. Enhancement

This week is about enhancing and lifting your face and your mood. Using a tool such as a pencil is an easy way to help encourage both sides of the face to work together, to add resistance and to help gain more control over what the muscles are doing.

TECHNIQUE OF THE WEEK
The Jaw Enhancing Technique

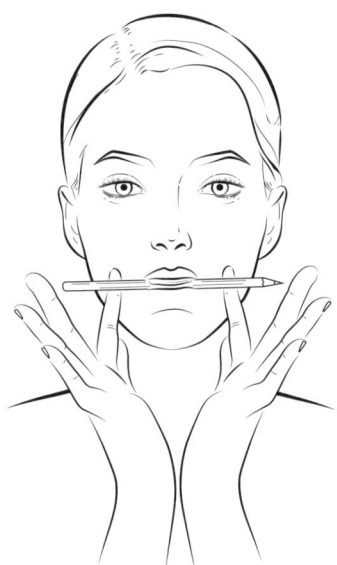

1. Place a pencil horizontally in your mouth, behind your canine teeth. Gently grip it with your teeth. Use your index fingers to smooth any creases by the cheeks. Gently tilt your head back as far as is comfortable and hold for 10 seconds, feeling the jaw muscles engage.

2. Relax and take a break, then repeat as many times as feels right for you, doing a maximum of 10 repetitions.

Benefits: This technique enhances the jawline by toning many of the lower face muscles. As the muscles build in strength and tone with daily practice, the lower face appears smoother, firmer and more lifted.

> **Weekly wellness hack** This week is about enhancing and lifting your mood. Ring a friend or family member and talk about how you really feel – whether you feel happy or sad. Either way, it will be healing for you and they will feel pleased you have shared with them. Plus, if they are feeling the same, they won't feel as alone.

My Positive Word for the Week:

....

The Way I Want to Feel this Week:

....

My Reason for Doing Face Yoga this Week:

....

"Life is sometimes really damn tough but so are you."

MONDAY

Today's intention:

....

When I did my Face Yoga today:

AM practice .... minutes   PM practice .... minutes

The areas I worked on today:

☐ Forehead   ☐ Eyes   ☐ Cheeks   ☐ Mouth   ☐ Jaw   ☐ Neck   ☐ Wellness

What I am most grateful for today:

....

....

TUESDAY

Today's intention:

....

When I did my Face Yoga today:

AM practice .... minutes   PM practice .... minutes

The areas I worked on today:

☐ Forehead   ☐ Eyes   ☐ Cheeks   ☐ Mouth   ☐ Jaw   ☐ Neck   ☐ Wellness

What I am most grateful for today:

....

....

WEDNESDAY

Today's intention:

....

When I did my Face Yoga today:

AM practice .... minutes   PM practice .... minutes

The areas I worked on today:

☐ Forehead ☐ Eyes ☐ Cheeks ☐ Mouth ☐ Jaw ☐ Neck ☐ Wellness

What I am most grateful for today:

....

....

THURSDAY

Today's intention:

....

When I did my Face Yoga today:

AM practice .... minutes   PM practice .... minutes

The areas I worked on today:

☐ Forehead ☐ Eyes ☐ Cheeks ☐ Mouth ☐ Jaw ☐ Neck ☐ Wellness

What I am most grateful for today:

....

....

FRIDAY

Today's intention:

....

When I did my Face Yoga today:

AM practice .... minutes   PM practice .... minutes

The areas I worked on today:

☐ Forehead   ☐ Eyes   ☐ Cheeks   ☐ Mouth   ☐ Jaw   ☐ Neck   ☐ Wellness

What I am most grateful for today:

....

....

SATURDAY

Today's intention:

....

When I did my Face Yoga today:

AM practice .... minutes   PM practice .... minutes

The areas I worked on today:

☐ Forehead   ☐ Eyes   ☐ Cheeks   ☐ Mouth   ☐ Jaw   ☐ Neck   ☐ Wellness

What I am most grateful for today:

....

....

SUNDAY

Today's intention:

....

When I did my Face Yoga today:

AM practice .... minutes   PM practice .... minutes

The areas I worked on today:

☐ Forehead   ☐ Eyes   ☐ Cheeks   ☐ Mouth   ☐ Jaw   ☐ Neck   ☐ Wellness

What I am most grateful for today:

....

....

What Went Well this Week:

....

....

What Didn't Go so Well this Week:

....

....

Week 33. Empowerment

Prepare to feel empowered this week! One of the best ways to feel empowered is to create a sense of achievement by increasing your dopamine levels. Ticking off your daily Face Yoga, practising techniques such as the one this week where you instantly feel the muscles working, and even this week's wellness hack to sort out your finances, can all help with that dopamine hit and overall feeling of empowerment.

TECHNIQUE OF THE WEEK
The Neck Empowering Technique

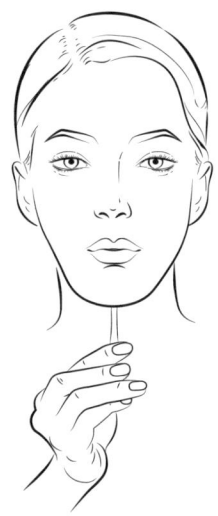

1. Making sure your chin is parallel to the floor and you have good posture, place the back of a teaspoon under your chin. Close your lips, breathe through your nose and keep your jaw relaxed. Press the spoon up into your chin and slightly lower your chin to create more resistance, as if your chin is trying to come down toward your chest but the spoon is stopping it.

2. Keep this for up to 1 minute.

Benefits: This is great for toning and lifting the area which is often prone to "turkey neck" or double chin. It's a simple technique but feels empowering to do daily to maintain muscle tone, posture and control over this area.

> **Weekly wellness hack** Good financial management is an important aspect of wellbeing and can help you feel empowered in all areas of your life. If you are able to, make it a priority this week to look at what money you can save, invest and spend, and even set aside some time to make a budgeting plan.

My Positive Word for the Week:

....

The Way I Want to Feel this Week:

....

My Reason for Doing Face Yoga this Week:

....

"Showing weakness doesn't make you any less strong; in fact, it can empower you."

MONDAY

Today's intention:

....

When I did my Face Yoga today:

AM practice .... minutes   PM practice .... minutes

The areas I worked on today:

☐ Forehead ☐ Eyes ☐ Cheeks ☐ Mouth ☐ Jaw ☐ Neck ☐ Wellness

What I am most grateful for today:

....

....

TUESDAY

Today's intention:

....

When I did my Face Yoga today:

AM practice .... minutes   PM practice .... minutes

The areas I worked on today:

☐ Forehead ☐ Eyes ☐ Cheeks ☐ Mouth ☐ Jaw ☐ Neck ☐ Wellness

What I am most grateful for today:

....

....

WEDNESDAY

Today's intention:

....

When I did my Face Yoga today:

AM practice .... minutes   PM practice .... minutes

The areas I worked on today:

☐ Forehead ☐ Eyes ☐ Cheeks ☐ Mouth ☐ Jaw ☐ Neck ☐ Wellness

What I am most grateful for today:

....

....

THURSDAY

Today's intention:

....

When I did my Face Yoga today:

AM practice .... minutes   PM practice .... minutes

The areas I worked on today:

☐ Forehead ☐ Eyes ☐ Cheeks ☐ Mouth ☐ Jaw ☐ Neck ☐ Wellness

What I am most grateful for today:

....

....

FRIDAY

Today's intention:

....

When I did my Face Yoga today:

AM practice .... minutes   PM practice .... minutes

The areas I worked on today:

☐ Forehead   ☐ Eyes   ☐ Cheeks   ☐ Mouth   ☐ Jaw   ☐ Neck   ☐ Wellness

What I am most grateful for today:

....

....

SATURDAY

Today's intention:

....

When I did my Face Yoga today:

AM practice .... minutes   PM practice .... minutes

The areas I worked on today:

☐ Forehead   ☐ Eyes   ☐ Cheeks   ☐ Mouth   ☐ Jaw   ☐ Neck   ☐ Wellness

What I am most grateful for today:

....

....

SUNDAY

Today's intention:

....

When I did my Face Yoga today:

AM practice .... minutes   PM practice .... minutes

The areas I worked on today:

☐ Forehead   ☐ Eyes   ☐ Cheeks   ☐ Mouth   ☐ Jaw   ☐ Neck   ☐ Wellness

What I am most grateful for today:

....

....

What Went Well this Week:

....

....

What Didn't Go so Well this Week:

....

....

Week 34. Smoothing

Smooth, lifted skin comes from a balance between strong toning moves and soft relaxing moves. This week is focused on the latter and the Face Yoga technique is designed to smooth the forehead. Another wonderful way to promote smooth skin is through breath, which has been proven in multiple studies to ease tension and strain in the face.

TECHNIQUE OF THE WEEK
The Forehead Smoothing Technique

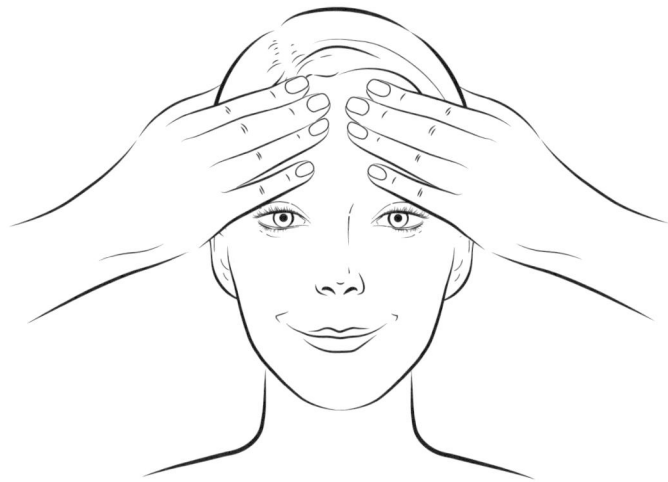

1. Place your little fingers over your eyebrows so that they fully cover each eyebrow, ensuring they stay smooth, and the rest of the fingers on your forehead, using them to keep the forehead as smooth as possible. Open your eyes wide without raising your eyebrows, take 3 deep breaths and repeat 3 times: "My forehead is smooth."

2. Relax, then do this once more.

Benefits: This is a beautiful way to smooth your forehead and prevent wrinkles. It will also soften existing lines and strengthen the eye muscles. The combination of the facial exercise and the affirmation can help to build a mind-muscle connection; they train your face to express with your eyes and not your forehead.

> **Weekly wellness hack** At the start of the week, take a few moments to make a sacred space in your home – it can be a small corner, table or even a whole room. Fill the space with things that help you feel calm, happy and grateful. Each day this week sit there for a few minutes and simply breathe.

My Positive Word for the Week:

....

The Way I Want to Feel this Week:

....

My Reason for Doing Face Yoga this Week:

....

"Do one thing each day, however tiny it may be, which makes you feel like you are alive."

MONDAY

Today's intention:

....

When I did my Face Yoga today:

AM practice .... minutes   PM practice .... minutes

The areas I worked on today:

☐ Forehead ☐ Eyes ☐ Cheeks ☐ Mouth ☐ Jaw ☐ Neck ☐ Wellness

What I am most grateful for today:

....

....

TUESDAY

Today's intention:

....

When I did my Face Yoga today:

AM practice .... minutes   PM practice .... minutes

The areas I worked on today:

☐ Forehead ☐ Eyes ☐ Cheeks ☐ Mouth ☐ Jaw ☐ Neck ☐ Wellness

What I am most grateful for today:

....

....

WEDNESDAY

Today's intention:

....

When I did my Face Yoga today:

AM practice .... minutes   PM practice .... minutes

The areas I worked on today:

☐ Forehead   ☐ Eyes   ☐ Cheeks   ☐ Mouth   ☐ Jaw   ☐ Neck   ☐ Wellness

What I am most grateful for today:

....

....

THURSDAY

Today's intention:

....

When I did my Face Yoga today:

AM practice .... minutes   PM practice .... minutes

The areas I worked on today:

☐ Forehead   ☐ Eyes   ☐ Cheeks   ☐ Mouth   ☐ Jaw   ☐ Neck   ☐ Wellness

What I am most grateful for today:

....

....

FRIDAY

Today's intention:

....

When I did my Face Yoga today:

AM practice .... minutes   PM practice .... minutes

The areas I worked on today:

☐ Forehead   ☐ Eyes   ☐ Cheeks   ☐ Mouth   ☐ Jaw   ☐ Neck   ☐ Wellness

What I am most grateful for today:

....

....

SATURDAY

Today's intention:

....

When I did my Face Yoga today:

AM practice .... minutes   PM practice .... minutes

The areas I worked on today:

☐ Forehead   ☐ Eyes   ☐ Cheeks   ☐ Mouth   ☐ Jaw   ☐ Neck   ☐ Wellness

What I am most grateful for today:

....

....

SUNDAY

Today's intention:

....

When I did my Face Yoga today:

AM practice .... minutes   PM practice .... minutes

The areas I worked on today:

☐ Forehead ☐ Eyes ☐ Cheeks ☐ Mouth ☐ Jaw ☐ Neck ☐ Wellness

What I am most grateful for today:

....

....

What Went Well this Week:

....

....

What Didn't Go so Well this Week:

....

....

Week 35. Radiating

This week is about radiating the best version of you. The Danielle Collins Face Yoga Method isn't about looking like someone else or even like your younger self; it's about looking amazing for your age, radiating confidence, glowing from the inside out and having smooth, lifted skin in the present moment.

TECHNIQUE OF THE WEEK
The Eye Radiating Technique

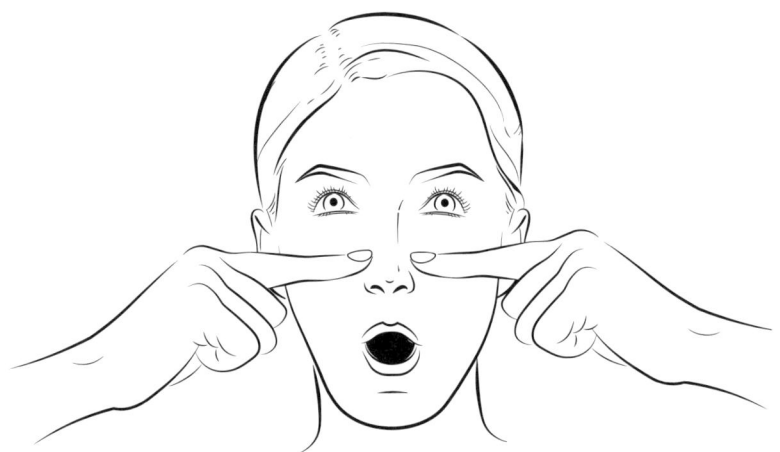

1. Make your mouth into an "O" shape and wrap your lips around your teeth. Using both hands, place your index fingers horizontally under your eyes where you feel your bone. Look up and flutter the upper eyelids. Continue for 30 seconds.

2. Take a break and repeat a second time.

Benefits: This technique is amazing for reducing hollows under your eyes, firming the eyelids and brightening the eyes so they radiate energy. It also lifts and tones the area around the mouth.

Weekly wellness hack One of the best ways to radiate energy, calm and positivity is to do daily affirmations. Start your affirmation with "I am…" and add any helpful words or phrases that represent the way you would like to feel, look or be. It can be anything that resonates with you.

My Positive Word for the Week:

....

The Way I Want to Feel this Week:

....

My Reason for Doing Face Yoga this Week:

....

"Radiate out the energy you want to receive back."

MONDAY

Today's intention:

....

When I did my Face Yoga today:

AM practice .... minutes   PM practice .... minutes

The areas I worked on today:

☐ Forehead ☐ Eyes ☐ Cheeks ☐ Mouth ☐ Jaw ☐ Neck ☐ Wellness

What I am most grateful for today:

....

....

TUESDAY

Today's intention:

....

When I did my Face Yoga today:

AM practice .... minutes   PM practice .... minutes

The areas I worked on today:

☐ Forehead ☐ Eyes ☐ Cheeks ☐ Mouth ☐ Jaw ☐ Neck ☐ Wellness

What I am most grateful for today:

....

....

WEDNESDAY

Today's intention:

....

When I did my Face Yoga today:

AM practice .... minutes   PM practice .... minutes

The areas I worked on today:

☐ Forehead ☐ Eyes ☐ Cheeks ☐ Mouth ☐ Jaw ☐ Neck ☐ Wellness

What I am most grateful for today:

....

....

THURSDAY

Today's intention:

....

When I did my Face Yoga today:

AM practice .... minutes   PM practice .... minutes

The areas I worked on today:

☐ Forehead ☐ Eyes ☐ Cheeks ☐ Mouth ☐ Jaw ☐ Neck ☐ Wellness

What I am most grateful for today:

....

....

FRIDAY

Today's intention:

....

When I did my Face Yoga today:

AM practice .... minutes   PM practice .... minutes

The areas I worked on today:

☐ Forehead ☐ Eyes ☐ Cheeks ☐ Mouth ☐ Jaw ☐ Neck ☐ Wellness

What I am most grateful for today:

....

....

SATURDAY

Today's intention:

....

When I did my Face Yoga today:

AM practice .... minutes   PM practice .... minutes

The areas I worked on today:

☐ Forehead ☐ Eyes ☐ Cheeks ☐ Mouth ☐ Jaw ☐ Neck ☐ Wellness

What I am most grateful for today:

....

....

SUNDAY

Today's intention:

....

When I did my Face Yoga today:

AM practice .... minutes   PM practice .... minutes

The areas I worked on today:

☐ Forehead ☐ Eyes ☐ Cheeks ☐ Mouth ☐ Jaw ☐ Neck ☐ Wellness

What I am most grateful for today:

....

....

What Went Well this Week:

....

....

What Didn't Go so Well this Week:

....

....

Week 36. Strength

Strengthening facial muscles, particularly around the cheek area, is key for a youthful look. A BBC conducted a study where a doctor used The Danielle Collins Face Yoga Method and was analysed with a high-tech skin machine. It showed that Face Yoga can make you look 1 year younger in 4 weeks with 30 minutes practice per day. By now you may be in a regular routine of around 30 minutes.

The Cheek Strengthening Technique

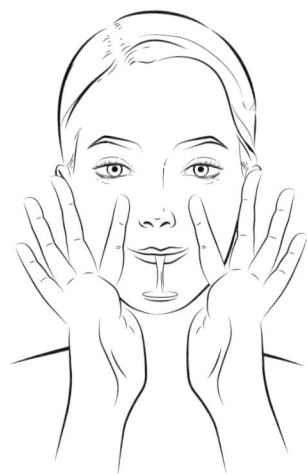

1. Place the end of a clean teaspoon in your mouth with your lips tucked in and the corners of your mouth lifted up. Using both hands, place your index fingers on the nasolabial folds and use them to smooth any lines created and to add some resistance. Move the spoon up and down 10 times, then take it out and relax.

2. Repeat twice more.

3. Close your eyes and relax your mouth and face for 30 seconds.

Benefits: This is a deeply strengthening technique for the muscles in the cheek area, mouth and jaw. It helps lift and firm sagging skin on the cheeks.

> **Weekly wellness hack** One of the best ways to feel inner strength in mind and body is to start to be aware of the negative voice we often use toward ourselves. You don't need to fight it or even try to change it at first; simply start by being an observer looking in and notice what words you use when you look in the mirror, feel sad or unwell. Awareness is strength.

My Positive Word for the Week:

....

The Way I Want to Feel this Week:

....

My Reason for Doing Face Yoga this Week:

....

"We are always stronger when we uplift each other."

MONDAY

Today's intention:

....

When I did my Face Yoga today:

AM practice .... minutes   PM practice .... minutes

The areas I worked on today:

☐ Forehead ☐ Eyes ☐ Cheeks ☐ Mouth ☐ Jaw ☐ Neck ☐ Wellness

What I am most grateful for today:

....

....

TUESDAY

Today's intention:

....

When I did my Face Yoga today:

AM practice .... minutes   PM practice .... minutes

The areas I worked on today:

☐ Forehead ☐ Eyes ☐ Cheeks ☐ Mouth ☐ Jaw ☐ Neck ☐ Wellness

What I am most grateful for today:

....

....

WEDNESDAY

Today's intention:

....

When I did my Face Yoga today:

AM practice .... minutes   PM practice .... minutes

The areas I worked on today:

☐ Forehead ☐ Eyes ☐ Cheeks ☐ Mouth ☐ Jaw ☐ Neck ☐ Wellness

What I am most grateful for today:

....

....

THURSDAY

Today's intention:

....

When I did my Face Yoga today:

AM practice .... minutes   PM practice .... minutes

The areas I worked on today:

☐ Forehead ☐ Eyes ☐ Cheeks ☐ Mouth ☐ Jaw ☐ Neck ☐ Wellness

What I am most grateful for today:

....

....

FRIDAY

Today's intention:

....

When I did my Face Yoga today:

AM practice .... minutes   PM practice .... minutes

The areas I worked on today:

☐ Forehead ☐ Eyes ☐ Cheeks ☐ Mouth ☐ Jaw ☐ Neck ☐ Wellness

What I am most grateful for today:

....

....

SATURDAY

Today's intention:

....

When I did my Face Yoga today:

AM practice .... minutes   PM practice .... minutes

The areas I worked on today:

☐ Forehead ☐ Eyes ☐ Cheeks ☐ Mouth ☐ Jaw ☐ Neck ☐ Wellness

What I am most grateful for today:

....

....

SUNDAY

Today's intention:

....

When I did my Face Yoga today:

AM practice .... minutes   PM practice .... minutes

The areas I worked on today:

☐ Forehead ☐ Eyes ☐ Cheeks ☐ Mouth ☐ Jaw ☐ Neck ☐ Wellness

What I am most grateful for today:

....

....

What Went Well this Week:

....

....

What Didn't Go so Well this Week:

....

....

Week 37. Alignment

Aligning ourselves has many meanings. Tuning in to your third eye chakra with meditation, crystals or the colour indigo can help you to tap into your intuition and feel aligned with your true self. Music and sound is another wonderful way to do this, as is knowing when to say no and when to say yes. Alignment of the face helps it to appear more youthful and attractive – but know that it's very normal for the face to have asymmetry; no one is perfect!

TECHNIQUE OF THE WEEK
The Mouth Aligning Technique

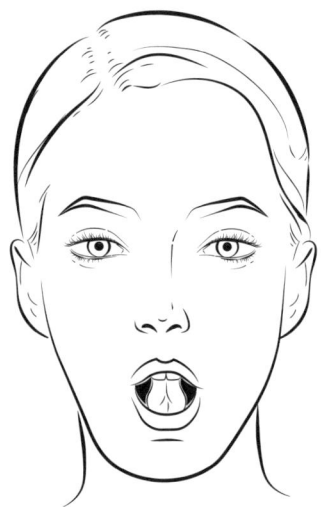

1. Make your mouth into an "O" shape and very slightly curl in the lips, but not with too much tension. Push the tip of your tongue back toward your tonsils. Then push it toward one cheek, then toward the other without actually touching either cheek with the tongue.

2. Keep repeating the sequence for 1 minute, using a mirror to ensure you move the tongue equally to each side.

Benefits: This helps to strengthen the muscles in the tongue and around the mouth, and helps bring symmetry to the mouth area. It's really useful to use a mirror to make sure you are working both sides equally. Never exercise through pain, so stop if it feels too strong or painful.

> **Weekly wellness hack** Find a relaxing sound that's in alignment with the way you want to feel each day this week. For example, it may be the real sounds of nature or a particular type of music. Notice how the power of sound can lift you and help you feel in alignment.

My Positive Word for the Week:

....

The Way I Want to Feel this Week:

....

My Reason for Doing Face Yoga this Week:

....

"Try saying 'no' more without the guilt. Try saying 'yes' more without the fear."

MONDAY

Today's intention:

....

When I did my Face Yoga today:

AM practice .... minutes　　PM practice .... minutes

The areas I worked on today:

☐ Forehead　☐ Eyes　☐ Cheeks　☐ Mouth　☐ Jaw　☐ Neck　☐ Wellness

What I am most grateful for today:

....

....

TUESDAY

Today's intention:

....

When I did my Face Yoga today:

AM practice .... minutes　　PM practice .... minutes

The areas I worked on today:

☐ Forehead　☐ Eyes　☐ Cheeks　☐ Mouth　☐ Jaw　☐ Neck　☐ Wellness

What I am most grateful for today:

....

....

WEDNESDAY

Today's intention:

....

When I did my Face Yoga today:

AM practice .... minutes   PM practice .... minutes

The areas I worked on today:

☐ Forehead ☐ Eyes ☐ Cheeks ☐ Mouth ☐ Jaw ☐ Neck ☐ Wellness

What I am most grateful for today:

....

....

THURSDAY

Today's intention:

....

When I did my Face Yoga today:

AM practice .... minutes   PM practice .... minutes

The areas I worked on today:

☐ Forehead ☐ Eyes ☐ Cheeks ☐ Mouth ☐ Jaw ☐ Neck ☐ Wellness

What I am most grateful for today:

....

....

FRIDAY

Today's intention:

....

When I did my Face Yoga today:

AM practice .... minutes   PM practice .... minutes

The areas I worked on today:

☐ Forehead ☐ Eyes ☐ Cheeks ☐ Mouth ☐ Jaw ☐ Neck ☐ Wellness

What I am most grateful for today:

....

....

SATURDAY

Today's intention:

....

When I did my Face Yoga today:

AM practice .... minutes   PM practice .... minutes

The areas I worked on today:

☐ Forehead ☐ Eyes ☐ Cheeks ☐ Mouth ☐ Jaw ☐ Neck ☐ Wellness

What I am most grateful for today:

....

....

SUNDAY

Today's intention:

....

When I did my Face Yoga today:

AM practice .... minutes   PM practice .... minutes

The areas I worked on today:

☐ Forehead   ☐ Eyes   ☐ Cheeks   ☐ Mouth   ☐ Jaw   ☐ Neck   ☐ Wellness

What I am most grateful for today:

....

....

What Went Well this Week:

....

....

What Didn't Go so Well this Week:

....

....

Week 38. Illumination

Time to illuminate! This word instantly makes us feel alive and full of light. This week your focus should be on the concept of illumination. Your Face Yoga will really help the skin to look lifted and illuminated, and using the seasonal mantra "I see, trust and know my own inner and outer beauty" will help the mind feel this way too.

TECHNIQUE OF THE WEEK
The Jaw Illuminating Technique

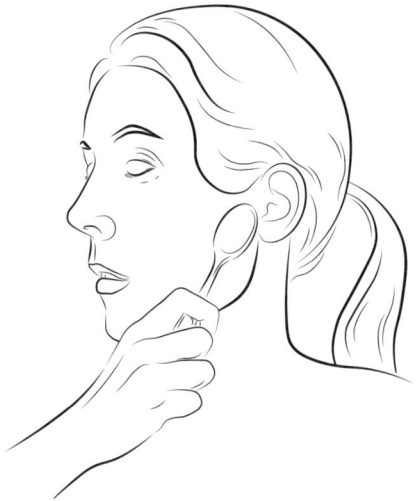

1. Apply your serum or oil to a clean face. Place the back of a cold teaspoon (ideally from the fridge) on your chin. With gentle pressure, smooth up your jawline, just above the bone, to the top of the ear. Lift off and go back to the starting position.

2. Repeat 30 times, only moving upward.

3. Repeat on the other side.

Benefits: This lifting and cooling massage helps to boost circulation, reduce puffiness and inflammation and release tension from tight jaw muscles.

Weekly wellness hack Take some time this week to write down three things that truly light you up. They should be things that make you feel like your true self and feel exciting yet grounding all at the same time. Acknowledging what these are is the first step to starting to do them more!

My Positive Word for the Week:

....

The Way I Want to Feel this Week:

....

My Reason for Doing Face Yoga this Week:

....

"Life is like a wave, a series of peaks and troughs, so let that wave flow."

MONDAY

Today's intention:

....

When I did my Face Yoga today:

AM practice .... minutes   PM practice .... minutes

The areas I worked on today:

☐ Forehead   ☐ Eyes   ☐ Cheeks   ☐ Mouth   ☐ Jaw   ☐ Neck   ☐ Wellness

What I am most grateful for today:

....

....

TUESDAY

Today's intention:

....

When I did my Face Yoga today:

AM practice .... minutes   PM practice .... minutes

The areas I worked on today:

☐ Forehead   ☐ Eyes   ☐ Cheeks   ☐ Mouth   ☐ Jaw   ☐ Neck   ☐ Wellness

What I am most grateful for today:

....

....

WEDNESDAY

Today's intention:

....

When I did my Face Yoga today:

AM practice .... minutes   PM practice .... minutes

The areas I worked on today:

☐ Forehead   ☐ Eyes   ☐ Cheeks   ☐ Mouth   ☐ Jaw   ☐ Neck   ☐ Wellness

What I am most grateful for today:

....

....

THURSDAY

Today's intention:

....

When I did my Face Yoga today:

AM practice .... minutes   PM practice .... minutes

The areas I worked on today:

☐ Forehead   ☐ Eyes   ☐ Cheeks   ☐ Mouth   ☐ Jaw   ☐ Neck   ☐ Wellness

What I am most grateful for today:

....

....

FRIDAY

Today's intention:

....

When I did my Face Yoga today:

AM practice .... minutes   PM practice .... minutes

The areas I worked on today:

☐ Forehead ☐ Eyes ☐ Cheeks ☐ Mouth ☐ Jaw ☐ Neck ☐ Wellness

What I am most grateful for today:

....

....

SATURDAY

Today's intention:

....

When I did my Face Yoga today:

AM practice .... minutes   PM practice .... minutes

The areas I worked on today:

☐ Forehead ☐ Eyes ☐ Cheeks ☐ Mouth ☐ Jaw ☐ Neck ☐ Wellness

What I am most grateful for today:

....

....

SUNDAY

Today's intention:

....

When I did my Face Yoga today:

AM practice .... minutes   PM practice .... minutes

The areas I worked on today:

☐ Forehead ☐ Eyes ☐ Cheeks ☐ Mouth ☐ Jaw ☐ Neck ☐ Wellness

What I am most grateful for today:

....

....

What Went Well this Week:

....

....

What Didn't Go so Well this Week:

....

....

Week 39. Toning

The most common area that people want to tone is the neck. The major muscle in the neck, the platysma, is a broad sheet of muscle that runs all the way from the collarbone to the jawline. The skin on the neck is very thin (the second thinnest of the whole body, after the eye area) and as we age the platysma loses fat and muscle tone. This week is about gently lifting and toning the neck and the wellness hack is about toning the skin on the rest of the body too.

The Neck Toning Technique

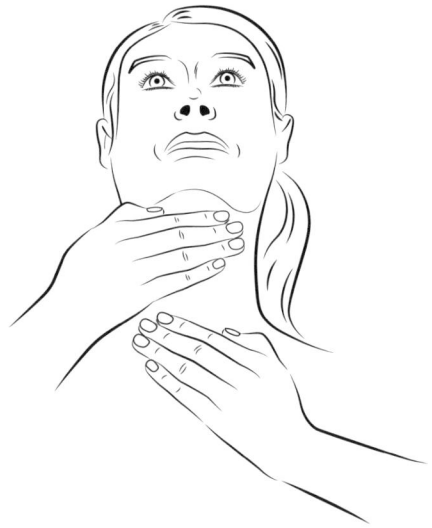

1. Gently tilt your head back as far as is comfortable for you and place one hand under the chin and one on the collarbone. Silently and slowly say the word "Yum".

2. Repeat and continue for 1 minute.

Benefits: This lifts and tones the muscles in the neck, jaw and mouth and therefore firms the skin and smooths lines.

> **Weekly wellness hack** This week is all about toning the skin on your body. Before every shower or bath, dry body brush, with long strokes toward the heart, to improve circulation, energy, and reduce cellulite. Follow each shower or bath with a full-body moisturize for hydration.

My Positive Word for the Week:

....

The Way I Want to Feel this Week:

....

My Reason for Doing Face Yoga this Week:

....

"We have two choices. We can focus on what we have. Or we can focus on what's missing."

MONDAY

Today's intention:

....

When I did my Face Yoga today:

AM practice .... minutes   PM practice .... minutes

The areas I worked on today:

☐ Forehead ☐ Eyes ☐ Cheeks ☐ Mouth ☐ Jaw ☐ Neck ☐ Wellness

What I am most grateful for today:

....

....

TUESDAY

Today's intention:

....

When I did my Face Yoga today:

AM practice .... minutes   PM practice .... minutes

The areas I worked on today:

☐ Forehead ☐ Eyes ☐ Cheeks ☐ Mouth ☐ Jaw ☐ Neck ☐ Wellness

What I am most grateful for today:

....

....

WEDNESDAY

Today's intention:

....

When I did my Face Yoga today:

AM practice .... minutes   PM practice .... minutes

The areas I worked on today:

☐ Forehead ☐ Eyes ☐ Cheeks ☐ Mouth ☐ Jaw ☐ Neck ☐ Wellness

What I am most grateful for today:

....

....

THURSDAY

Today's intention:

....

When I did my Face Yoga today:

AM practice .... minutes   PM practice .... minutes

The areas I worked on today:

☐ Forehead ☐ Eyes ☐ Cheeks ☐ Mouth ☐ Jaw ☐ Neck ☐ Wellness

What I am most grateful for today:

....

....

FRIDAY

Today's intention:

....

When I did my Face Yoga today:

AM practice .... minutes   PM practice .... minutes

The areas I worked on today:

☐ Forehead ☐ Eyes ☐ Cheeks ☐ Mouth ☐ Jaw ☐ Neck ☐ Wellness

What I am most grateful for today:

....

....

SATURDAY

Today's intention:

....

When I did my Face Yoga today:

AM practice .... minutes   PM practice .... minutes

The areas I worked on today:

☐ Forehead ☐ Eyes ☐ Cheeks ☐ Mouth ☐ Jaw ☐ Neck ☐ Wellness

What I am most grateful for today:

....

....

SUNDAY

Today's intention:

....

When I did my Face Yoga today:

AM practice .... minutes   PM practice .... minutes

The areas I worked on today:

☐ Forehead   ☐ Eyes   ☐ Cheeks   ☐ Mouth   ☐ Jaw   ☐ Neck   ☐ Wellness

What I am most grateful for today:

....

....

What Went Well this Week:

....

....

What Didn't Go so Well this Week:

....

....

Season 4
Soothe your face

Happiness chemical: serotonin
Chakras: root chakra and throat chakra
Crystals: black tourmaline and turquoise
Colours: red and blue

Mantra: "I speak words that resonate with who I truly am."

You have reached your final season, which is such an amazing achievement, so firstly take a moment to feel proud (which will also release this season's happiness chemical, serotonin!).

This season is all about soothing the face, mind and body. There is now an evidenced-based branch of medicine called psychodermatology that's championed by the British Association of Dermatologists, which connects our emotions to the health of our skin and vice versa. Soothing the face and all that comes with it from an aesthetic point of view (clear, glowing, smooth skin) is also about learning to acknowledge and release stress. This season we focus on two chakras, the first being the root chakra, which is connected to a feeling of being grounded. We can balance this chakra through the colour red and our black tourmaline crystal. All the techniques, wellness hacks and positive statements this season will help you develop this feeling of being rooted and in touch with your body; therefore, they all help to ease stress.

The second chakra of this season is the throat chakra, which is balanced and soothed by the colour blue and the crystal turquoise. The throat chakra is connected to speaking our truth and tuning in to our authentic voice. My hope is that over the past nine months all the activities and techniques in this journal have helped you already with this; I hope that you have a better understanding of what you truly want and who you truly are. If you feel this is something you could work on more, this season is your chance to do it. Starting with using the seasonal mantra, "I speak words that resonate with who I truly am", will help.

All the weekly themes over this final season help to soothe your face. This is all about gentle loving care to help your skin look and feel wonderful.

Week 40. Cherishing

To start this soothing season, you are going to cherish yourself through gentle facial touch and rest. Your turquoise crystal is wonderful to have around you this week to help cherish your authentic voice.

The Face Cherishing Technique

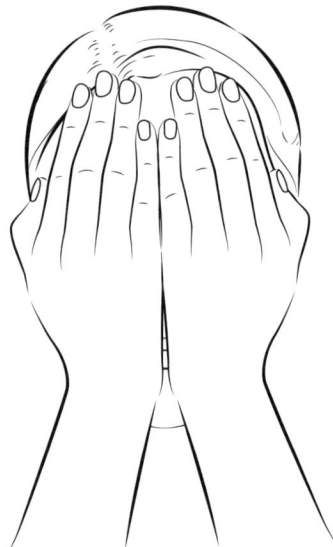

1. Rub your hands together for 20 seconds to build up warmth.

2. Cup your hands lightly over your face for 40 seconds and breathe deeply, feeling a sense of cherishing your skin as the warmth and energy release tension from your muscles.

Benefits: Rubbing your hands together increases the *prana* or *qi*. This is then transferred to your face, which not only helps the face to look healthier but you will feel stress melting away as you touch and breathe.

> **Weekly wellness hack** This week, cherish the power of rest and spend a little extra time in bed. Ideally go to bed early but you could also lie in or take an afternoon nap. Enjoy the extra rest and time alone.

My Positive Word for the Week:

....

The Way I Want to Feel this Week:

....

My Reason for Doing Face Yoga this Week:

....

"You are special. Cherish that."

MONDAY

Today's intention:

....

When I did my Face Yoga today:

AM practice .... minutes   PM practice .... minutes

The areas I worked on today:

☐ Forehead   ☐ Eyes   ☐ Cheeks   ☐ Mouth   ☐ Jaw   ☐ Neck   ☐ Wellness

What I am most grateful for today:

....

....

TUESDAY

Today's intention:

....

When I did my Face Yoga today:

AM practice .... minutes   PM practice .... minutes

The areas I worked on today:

☐ Forehead   ☐ Eyes   ☐ Cheeks   ☐ Mouth   ☐ Jaw   ☐ Neck   ☐ Wellness

What I am most grateful for today:

....

....

WEDNESDAY

Today's intention:

....

When I did my Face Yoga today:

AM practice .... minutes   PM practice .... minutes

The areas I worked on today:

☐ Forehead   ☐ Eyes   ☐ Cheeks   ☐ Mouth   ☐ Jaw   ☐ Neck   ☐ Wellness

What I am most grateful for today:

....

....

THURSDAY

Today's intention:

....

When I did my Face Yoga today:

AM practice .... minutes   PM practice .... minutes

The areas I worked on today:

☐ Forehead   ☐ Eyes   ☐ Cheeks   ☐ Mouth   ☐ Jaw   ☐ Neck   ☐ Wellness

What I am most grateful for today:

....

....

FRIDAY

Today's intention:

....

When I did my Face Yoga today:

AM practice .... minutes   PM practice .... minutes

The areas I worked on today:

☐ Forehead ☐ Eyes ☐ Cheeks ☐ Mouth ☐ Jaw ☐ Neck ☐ Wellness

What I am most grateful for today:

....

....

SATURDAY

Today's intention:

....

When I did my Face Yoga today:

AM practice .... minutes   PM practice .... minutes

The areas I worked on today:

☐ Forehead ☐ Eyes ☐ Cheeks ☐ Mouth ☐ Jaw ☐ Neck ☐ Wellness

What I am most grateful for today:

....

....

SUNDAY

Today's intention:

....

When I did my Face Yoga today:

AM practice .... minutes   PM practice .... minutes

The areas I worked on today:

☐ Forehead   ☐ Eyes   ☐ Cheeks   ☐ Mouth   ☐ Jaw   ☐ Neck   ☐ Wellness

What I am most grateful for today:

....

....

What Went Well this Week:

....

....

What Didn't Go so Well this Week:

....

....

Week 41. Slowing

We often think that with many things in life, including our Face Yoga, going hard and fast gets better results. Very often the complete opposite is true. Being slow, gentle and mindful (where we focus on the present moment, the only place that we can truly feel at peace) very often makes our Face Yoga more effective because the skin responds better to this approach. Aim to see what you can slow down in your life this week and notice the benefits of this.

TECHNIQUE OF THE WEEK
The Forehead Slowing Technique

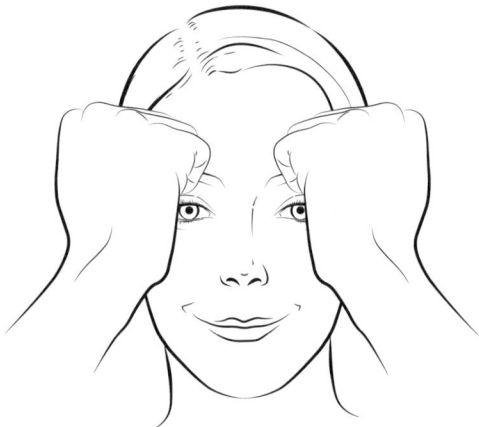

1. Make your hands into fists and place your finger joints so they are in line with your eyebrows. Using little circular motions, very slowly start to massage upward toward the hairline. Lift off and start from the eyebrows again.

2. Continue slowly for 1 minute whilst breathing deeply.

Benefits: With this technique you are slowly yet effectively working the fascia, which is the connective tissue under skin. As we release tension and improve circulation in the fascia, the skin looks healthier and lines appear smoother.

> **Weekly wellness hack** Each time you eat this week, take some time to chew every mouthful slowly. This is better for your digestion – and therefore your skin – but it's also a mindfulness practice that soothes and calms the mind.

My Positive Word for the Week:

....

The Way I Want to Feel this Week:

....

My Reason for Doing Face Yoga this Week:

....

"It's okay to go slow and still reach your goals."

MONDAY

Today's intention:

....

When I did my Face Yoga today:

AM practice .... minutes   PM practice .... minutes

The areas I worked on today:

☐ Forehead ☐ Eyes ☐ Cheeks ☐ Mouth ☐ Jaw ☐ Neck ☐ Wellness

What I am most grateful for today:

....

....

TUESDAY

Today's intention:

....

When I did my Face Yoga today:

AM practice .... minutes   PM practice .... minutes

The areas I worked on today:

☐ Forehead ☐ Eyes ☐ Cheeks ☐ Mouth ☐ Jaw ☐ Neck ☐ Wellness

What I am most grateful for today:

....

....

WEDNESDAY

Today's intention:

....

When I did my Face Yoga today:

AM practice .... minutes   PM practice .... minutes

The areas I worked on today:

☐ Forehead ☐ Eyes ☐ Cheeks ☐ Mouth ☐ Jaw ☐ Neck ☐ Wellness

What I am most grateful for today:

....

....

THURSDAY

Today's intention:

....

When I did my Face Yoga today:

AM practice .... minutes   PM practice .... minutes

The areas I worked on today:

☐ Forehead ☐ Eyes ☐ Cheeks ☐ Mouth ☐ Jaw ☐ Neck ☐ Wellness

What I am most grateful for today:

....

....

FRIDAY

Today's intention:

....

When I did my Face Yoga today:

AM practice .... minutes   PM practice .... minutes

The areas I worked on today:

☐ Forehead ☐ Eyes ☐ Cheeks ☐ Mouth ☐ Jaw ☐ Neck ☐ Wellness

What I am most grateful for today:

....

....

SATURDAY

Today's intention:

....

When I did my Face Yoga today:

AM practice .... minutes   PM practice .... minutes

The areas I worked on today:

☐ Forehead ☐ Eyes ☐ Cheeks ☐ Mouth ☐ Jaw ☐ Neck ☐ Wellness

What I am most grateful for today:

....

....

SUNDAY

Today's intention:

....

When I did my Face Yoga today:

AM practice .... minutes   PM practice .... minutes

The areas I worked on today:

☐ Forehead   ☐ Eyes   ☐ Cheeks   ☐ Mouth   ☐ Jaw   ☐ Neck   ☐ Wellness

What I am most grateful for today:

....

....

What Went Well this Week:

....

....

What Didn't Go so Well this Week:

....

....

Week 42. Clearing

This week's Face Yoga and wellness hacks are about clearing. When there is a blockage in the lymphatic system (the system in the body which carries white blood cells for immunity and helps remove bodily waste), fluid can build up. In the face this can show as puffiness, dark circles, uneven skin, spots and bloating. Your Face Yoga technique this week stimulates the lymphatic system. Have your black tourmaline crystal near you to further help the sense of clearing.

TECHNIQUE OF THE WEEK

The Eyes Clearing Technique

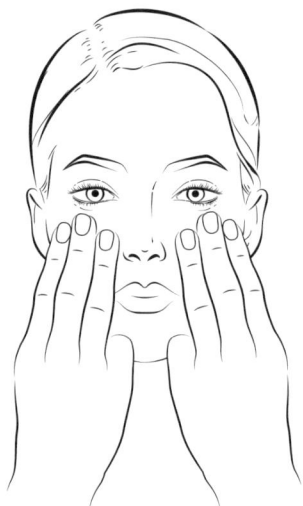

1. Using both hands, place your three fingertips under both eyes and very gently do little pulses on the skin. You want to be pressing so lightly that it is just skin, not muscle, you feel.

2. Continue this pulsing, moving outward toward the temples after each pulse, then slowly pulse down the side of the face and neck to the collarbone. The whole sequence should take around 1 minute.

Benefits: This helps with lymphatic drainage, which is great for glowing skin, reducing under-eye puffiness and bloating in the face. It is also a gentle, soothing massage for acne-prone skin because it can brighten the skin and aid detoxification.

> **Weekly wellness hack** For clear skin, get into the habit of cleaning your phone daily, changing your pillowcase every other day and also keeping your hair clean (and if it's dirty, then keep it tied back from your face). This will help reduce and prevent spots.

My Positive Word for the Week:

....

The Way I Want to Feel this Week:

....

My Reason for Doing Face Yoga this Week:

....

"Striving for peace is so much nicer than striving for perfection."

MONDAY

Today's intention:

....

When I did my Face Yoga today:

AM practice .... minutes   PM practice .... minutes

The areas I worked on today:

☐ Forehead   ☐ Eyes   ☐ Cheeks   ☐ Mouth   ☐ Jaw   ☐ Neck   ☐ Wellness

What I am most grateful for today:

....

....

TUESDAY

Today's intention:

....

When I did my Face Yoga today:

AM practice .... minutes   PM practice .... minutes

The areas I worked on today:

☐ Forehead   ☐ Eyes   ☐ Cheeks   ☐ Mouth   ☐ Jaw   ☐ Neck   ☐ Wellness

What I am most grateful for today:

....

....

WEDNESDAY

Today's intention:

....

When I did my Face Yoga today:

AM practice .... minutes   PM practice .... minutes

The areas I worked on today:

☐ Forehead ☐ Eyes ☐ Cheeks ☐ Mouth ☐ Jaw ☐ Neck ☐ Wellness

What I am most grateful for today:

....

....

THURSDAY

Today's intention:

....

When I did my Face Yoga today:

AM practice .... minutes   PM practice .... minutes

The areas I worked on today:

☐ Forehead ☐ Eyes ☐ Cheeks ☐ Mouth ☐ Jaw ☐ Neck ☐ Wellness

What I am most grateful for today:

....

....

FRIDAY

Today's intention:

....

When I did my Face Yoga today:

AM practice .... minutes　　PM practice .... minutes

The areas I worked on today:

☐ Forehead　☐ Eyes　☐ Cheeks　☐ Mouth　☐ Jaw　☐ Neck　☐ Wellness

What I am most grateful for today:

....

....

SATURDAY

Today's intention:

....

When I did my Face Yoga today:

AM practice .... minutes　　PM practice .... minutes

The areas I worked on today:

☐ Forehead　☐ Eyes　☐ Cheeks　☐ Mouth　☐ Jaw　☐ Neck　☐ Wellness

What I am most grateful for today:

....

....

SUNDAY

Today's intention:

....

When I did my Face Yoga today:

AM practice .... minutes   PM practice .... minutes

The areas I worked on today:

☐ Forehead ☐ Eyes ☐ Cheeks ☐ Mouth ☐ Jaw ☐ Neck ☐ Wellness

What I am most grateful for today:

....

....

What Went Well this Week:

....

....

What Didn't Go so Well this Week:

....

....

Week 43. Centring

This week combines the many meanings of "centring". The authenticity of being ourselves, the core of the body, the symmetry of the face and working with the middle or centre layer of the skin, the dermis. The dermis contains two essential proteins called collagen and elastin. As we age, these are broken down. Exercising and massaging these areas helps to build more of these proteins, which thickens the dermis and plumps up the face.

TECHNIQUE OF THE WEEK
The Cheek Centring Technique

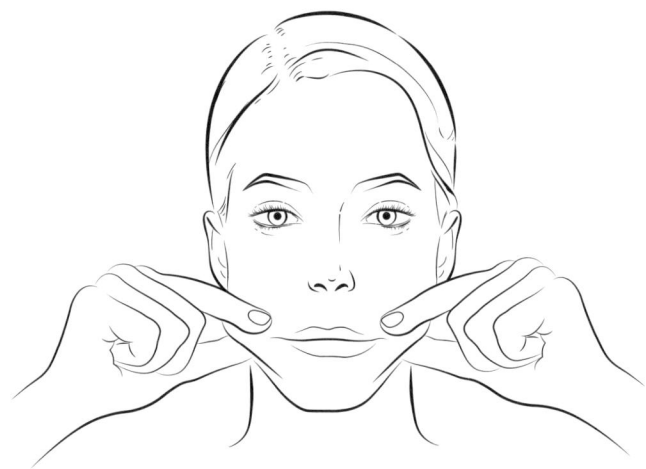

1. Using the index finger and thumb of one hand, gently squeeze the cheek muscles under the cheek bone. With your lips closed, smile slightly against the resistance. Use a mirror and ensure that you are using both sides of the face equally and that no lines are created whilst doing it.

2. Release the smile after 2 seconds, leaving the fingers where they are and continue doing up to 60 repetitions.

Benefits: This helps bring symmetry to the face by training both sides to be used equally. It can lift and firm the cheeks and helps the cheek area look healthier and glowing.

> **Weekly wellness hack** Focus on your core this week. This is your centre or "powerhouse". Doing core exercises, pilates or simply practising pulling in your pelvic floor and lower abdominal muscles then releasing them can help tone your centre.

My Positive Word for the Week:

....

The Way I Want to Feel this Week:

....

My Reason for Doing Face Yoga this Week:

....

"Deep down in your centre, at your very core, is the real you. You are always there."

MONDAY

Today's intention:

....

When I did my Face Yoga today:

AM practice .... minutes   PM practice .... minutes

The areas I worked on today:

☐ Forehead ☐ Eyes ☐ Cheeks ☐ Mouth ☐ Jaw ☐ Neck ☐ Wellness

What I am most grateful for today:

....

....

TUESDAY

Today's intention:

....

When I did my Face Yoga today:

AM practice .... minutes   PM practice .... minutes

The areas I worked on today:

☐ Forehead ☐ Eyes ☐ Cheeks ☐ Mouth ☐ Jaw ☐ Neck ☐ Wellness

What I am most grateful for today:

....

....

WEDNESDAY

Today's intention:

....

When I did my Face Yoga today:

AM practice .... minutes   PM practice .... minutes

The areas I worked on today:

☐ Forehead ☐ Eyes ☐ Cheeks ☐ Mouth ☐ Jaw ☐ Neck ☐ Wellness

What I am most grateful for today:

....

....

THURSDAY

Today's intention:

....

When I did my Face Yoga today:

AM practice .... minutes   PM practice .... minutes

The areas I worked on today:

☐ Forehead ☐ Eyes ☐ Cheeks ☐ Mouth ☐ Jaw ☐ Neck ☐ Wellness

What I am most grateful for today:

....

....

FRIDAY

Today's intention:

....

When I did my Face Yoga today:

AM practice .... minutes   PM practice .... minutes

The areas I worked on today:

☐ Forehead ☐ Eyes ☐ Cheeks ☐ Mouth ☐ Jaw ☐ Neck ☐ Wellness

What I am most grateful for today:

....

....

SATURDAY

Today's intention:

....

When I did my Face Yoga today:

AM practice .... minutes   PM practice .... minutes

The areas I worked on today:

☐ Forehead ☐ Eyes ☐ Cheeks ☐ Mouth ☐ Jaw ☐ Neck ☐ Wellness

What I am most grateful for today:

....

....

SUNDAY

Today's intention:

....

When I did my Face Yoga today:

AM practice .... minutes   PM practice .... minutes

The areas I worked on today:

☐ Forehead ☐ Eyes ☐ Cheeks ☐ Mouth ☐ Jaw ☐ Neck ☐ Wellness

What I am most grateful for today:

....

....

What Went Well this Week:

....

....

What Didn't Go so Well this Week:

....

....

Week 44. Admiration

As you approach the end of your year, my hope is that you are starting to feel a level of admiration for your skin, your mind and your body. As you do your Face Yoga technique, rather than focusing on the lines on your face, aim to massage out of a sense of admiration for your face and your efforts. Use your seasonal mantra as often as you can this week.

TECHNIQUE OF THE WEEK
The Mouth Admiring Technique

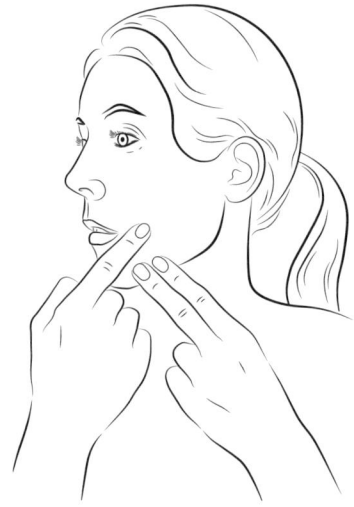

1. Apply serum or oil to your clean face. Place the pads of the index and middle fingers of your left hand on the left side of the jaw, directly below the left corner of your mouth. Using your right index finger, smooth the line from these fingers to your left nostril. Lift off and repeat again for 30 seconds.

2. Repeat on the other side for 30 seconds.

Benefits: This technique is great for smoothing and preventing marionette lines and smile lines. It also helps the skin to look brighter and feels very soothing.

Weekly wellness hack This may feel super difficult but it is so powerful. Stand naked in the mirror and say "I love you" three times. If emotions come up, just let them. But whatever happens, every day do this simple yet transformative activity.

My Positive Word for the Week:

....

The Way I Want to Feel this Week:

....

My Reason for Doing Face Yoga this Week:

....

"Do more things that make your heart feel beautiful."

MONDAY

Today's intention:

....

When I did my Face Yoga today:

AM practice .... minutes   PM practice .... minutes

The areas I worked on today:

☐ Forehead ☐ Eyes ☐ Cheeks ☐ Mouth ☐ Jaw ☐ Neck ☐ Wellness

What I am most grateful for today:

....

....

TUESDAY

Today's intention:

....

When I did my Face Yoga today:

AM practice .... minutes   PM practice .... minutes

The areas I worked on today:

☐ Forehead ☐ Eyes ☐ Cheeks ☐ Mouth ☐ Jaw ☐ Neck ☐ Wellness

What I am most grateful for today:

....

....

WEDNESDAY

Today's intention:

....

When I did my Face Yoga today:

AM practice .... minutes   PM practice .... minutes

The areas I worked on today:

☐ Forehead ☐ Eyes ☐ Cheeks ☐ Mouth ☐ Jaw ☐ Neck ☐ Wellness

What I am most grateful for today:

....

....

THURSDAY

Today's intention:

....

When I did my Face Yoga today:

AM practice .... minutes   PM practice .... minutes

The areas I worked on today:

☐ Forehead ☐ Eyes ☐ Cheeks ☐ Mouth ☐ Jaw ☐ Neck ☐ Wellness

What I am most grateful for today:

....

....

FRIDAY

Today's intention:

....

When I did my Face Yoga today:

AM practice .... minutes   PM practice .... minutes

The areas I worked on today:

☐ Forehead ☐ Eyes ☐ Cheeks ☐ Mouth ☐ Jaw ☐ Neck ☐ Wellness

What I am most grateful for today:

....

....

SATURDAY

Today's intention:

....

When I did my Face Yoga today:

AM practice .... minutes   PM practice .... minutes

The areas I worked on today:

☐ Forehead ☐ Eyes ☐ Cheeks ☐ Mouth ☐ Jaw ☐ Neck ☐ Wellness

What I am most grateful for today:

....

....

SUNDAY

Today's intention:

....

When I did my Face Yoga today:

AM practice .... minutes   PM practice .... minutes

The areas I worked on today:

☐ Forehead   ☐ Eyes   ☐ Cheeks   ☐ Mouth   ☐ Jaw   ☐ Neck   ☐ Wellness

What I am most grateful for today:

....

....

What Went Well this Week:

....

....

What Didn't Go so Well this Week:

....

....

Week 45. Elevation

This week's theme of elevation is about lifting and firming loose or sagging skin in the lower face, as well as helping yourself and others to feel great. Also take note of your posture whenever you sit this week. Imagine a string lifting you up from the top of your head, elevating you to the sky. At the same time, ground your root chakra by rooting your sit bones so you can feel them on the chair or floor. Great posture is the best elevation you can give yourself.

TECHNIQUE OF THE WEEK
The Jaw Elevating Technique

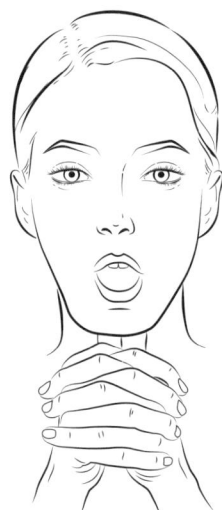

1. Link your fingers together and place the pads of both thumbs under your chin, making sure the thumbs are horizontal. Apply gentle pressure with the thumbs.

2. Use a mirror to ensure symmetry and gently open and close your mouth very slowly (a full open and close should take at least 10 seconds). Continue for 1 minute.

Benefits: This helps to elevate sagging skin under the chin by toning the underlying muscles around the jaw and neck. Because it's a slow, controlled movement it helps to train both sides of the lower face to work together equally as one, which can have a positive effect on facial alignment.

Weekly wellness hack This week do a random act of kindness to elevate happiness in others and yourself. Do something unexpected for someone you know or for a stranger, expecting nothing in return.

My Positive Word for the Week:

....

The Way I Want to Feel this Week:

....

My Reason for Doing Face Yoga this Week:

....

"Have belief in the seeds you are planting every day."

MONDAY

Today's intention:

....

When I did my Face Yoga today:

AM practice .... minutes   PM practice .... minutes

The areas I worked on today:

☐ Forehead ☐ Eyes ☐ Cheeks ☐ Mouth ☐ Jaw ☐ Neck ☐ Wellness

What I am most grateful for today:

....

....

TUESDAY

Today's intention:

....

When I did my Face Yoga today:

AM practice .... minutes   PM practice .... minutes

The areas I worked on today:

☐ Forehead ☐ Eyes ☐ Cheeks ☐ Mouth ☐ Jaw ☐ Neck ☐ Wellness

What I am most grateful for today:

....

....

WEDNESDAY

Today's intention:

....

When I did my Face Yoga today:

AM practice .... minutes   PM practice .... minutes

The areas I worked on today:

☐ Forehead ☐ Eyes ☐ Cheeks ☐ Mouth ☐ Jaw ☐ Neck ☐ Wellness

What I am most grateful for today:

....

....

THURSDAY

Today's intention:

....

When I did my Face Yoga today:

AM practice .... minutes   PM practice .... minutes

The areas I worked on today:

☐ Forehead ☐ Eyes ☐ Cheeks ☐ Mouth ☐ Jaw ☐ Neck ☐ Wellness

What I am most grateful for today:

....

....

FRIDAY

Today's intention:

....

When I did my Face Yoga today:

AM practice .... minutes   PM practice .... minutes

The areas I worked on today:

☐ Forehead ☐ Eyes ☐ Cheeks ☐ Mouth ☐ Jaw ☐ Neck ☐ Wellness

What I am most grateful for today:

....

....

SATURDAY

Today's intention:

....

When I did my Face Yoga today:

AM practice .... minutes   PM practice .... minutes

The areas I worked on today:

☐ Forehead ☐ Eyes ☐ Cheeks ☐ Mouth ☐ Jaw ☐ Neck ☐ Wellness

What I am most grateful for today:

....

....

SUNDAY

Today's intention:

....

When I did my Face Yoga today:

AM practice .... minutes   PM practice .... minutes

The areas I worked on today:

☐ Forehead ☐ Eyes ☐ Cheeks ☐ Mouth ☐ Jaw ☐ Neck ☐ Wellness

What I am most grateful for today:

....

....

What Went Well this Week:

....

....

What Didn't Go so Well this Week:

....

....

Week 46. Nourishment

Th is week is about nourishing your neck and shoulders, as well as your creativity and soul. Throughout the week, try to use your crystals, seasonal colours and mantra as much as you can. Also, focus on nourishing foods and drinking herbal teas. All of this will benefit your skin.

The Neck Nourishing Technique

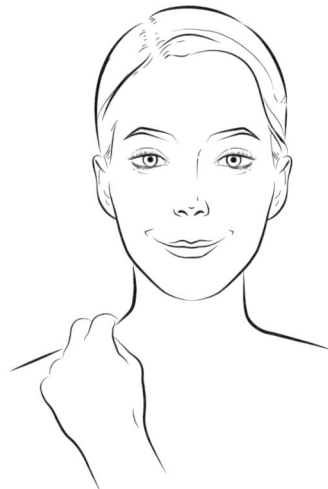

NOTE: This technique should be avoided if pregnant.

1. Find the spot halfway between your neck and your shoulder. It is often a little tender here so easy to find. Using one hand, place your index and middle fingers on that point and gently massage in a circular clockwise motion for around 15 seconds and anticlockwise for another 15 seconds.

2. With your other hand, repeat on the other shoulder. You can be quite intuitive in terms of pressure and speed.

Benefits: These nourishing acupressure points called Jian Jing or GB21 in Traditional Chinese Medicine are renowned for easing and soothing neck strain and neck and shoulder muscle tightness, and may ease headaches too.

Weekly wellness hack Enjoy the art of art this week to nourish your creativity. Spend some time looking at soothing and calming pictures online or, even better, at an art gallery. Notice how it allows you to be in the present moment and to just do something for the pure joy of it.

My Positive Word for the Week:

....

The Way I Want to Feel this Week:

....

My Reason for Doing Face Yoga this Week:

....

"Sometimes you need an inspirational statement to nourish your soul. Sometimes you need a hug, a movie and a cosy duvet day."

MONDAY

Today's intention:

....

When I did my Face Yoga today:

AM practice .... minutes   PM practice .... minutes

The areas I worked on today:

☐ Forehead ☐ Eyes ☐ Cheeks ☐ Mouth ☐ Jaw ☐ Neck ☐ Wellness

What I am most grateful for today:

....

....

TUESDAY

Today's intention:

....

When I did my Face Yoga today:

AM practice .... minutes   PM practice .... minutes

The areas I worked on today:

☐ Forehead ☐ Eyes ☐ Cheeks ☐ Mouth ☐ Jaw ☐ Neck ☐ Wellness

What I am most grateful for today:

....

....

WEDNESDAY

Today's intention:

....

When I did my Face Yoga today:

AM practice .... minutes   PM practice .... minutes

The areas I worked on today:

☐ Forehead   ☐ Eyes   ☐ Cheeks   ☐ Mouth   ☐ Jaw   ☐ Neck   ☐ Wellness

What I am most grateful for today:

....

....

THURSDAY

Today's intention:

....

When I did my Face Yoga today:

AM practice .... minutes   PM practice .... minutes

The areas I worked on today:

☐ Forehead   ☐ Eyes   ☐ Cheeks   ☐ Mouth   ☐ Jaw   ☐ Neck   ☐ Wellness

What I am most grateful for today:

....

....

FRIDAY

Today's intention:

....

When I did my Face Yoga today:

AM practice .... minutes   PM practice .... minutes

The areas I worked on today:

☐ Forehead   ☐ Eyes   ☐ Cheeks   ☐ Mouth   ☐ Jaw   ☐ Neck   ☐ Wellness

What I am most grateful for today:

....

....

SATURDAY

Today's intention:

....

When I did my Face Yoga today:

AM practice .... minutes   PM practice .... minutes

The areas I worked on today:

☐ Forehead   ☐ Eyes   ☐ Cheeks   ☐ Mouth   ☐ Jaw   ☐ Neck   ☐ Wellness

What I am most grateful for today:

....

....

SUNDAY

Today's intention:

....

When I did my Face Yoga today:

AM practice .... minutes   PM practice .... minutes

The areas I worked on today:

☐ Forehead   ☐ Eyes   ☐ Cheeks   ☐ Mouth   ☐ Jaw   ☐ Neck   ☐ Wellness

What I am most grateful for today:

....

....

What Went Well this Week:

....

....

What Didn't Go so Well this Week:

....

....

Week 47. Relaxation

Time to relax! By now you will know how Face Yoga and wellness can help you feel relaxed and studies confirm this. A Japanese study in 2018 showed that facial massage had a strong effect on stress alleviation, or psychological relaxation. A 2002 study showed the benefits of massage for easing headaches. It has also been shown that stress can be a factor causing acne (as well as a range of other skin disorders), and therefore relaxation is a key part of reducing this condition.

TECHNIQUE OF THE WEEK
The Forehead Relaxing Technique

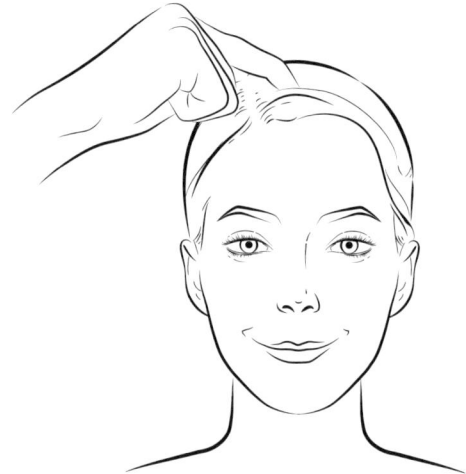

1. Measure two finger widths above your hairline and press one of your index fingers on this point, in the centre. It may feel a little tender so use light pressure at first. As you press this point focus on your breath and feel your forehead and head completely relaxing.

2. Continue holding for up to 1 minute.

Benefits: This point is renowned for easing headaches and for soothing stress and tension in the forehead, head and mind.

> **Weekly wellness hack** Invite some warmth into your week for utter relaxation. If it's sunny, spend some time outside. If not, use a hot water bottle, have a warm bath or drink warm tea. Do these warming rituals each day.

My Positive Word for the Week:

....

The Way I Want to Feel this Week:

....

My Reason for Doing Face Yoga this Week:

....

"Choose a day to relax your body completely now and again. If you don't, your body will choose one for you."

MONDAY

Today's intention:

....

When I did my Face Yoga today:

AM practice .... minutes   PM practice .... minutes

The areas I worked on today:

☐ Forehead ☐ Eyes ☐ Cheeks ☐ Mouth ☐ Jaw ☐ Neck ☐ Wellness

What I am most grateful for today:

....

....

TUESDAY

Today's intention:

....

When I did my Face Yoga today:

AM practice .... minutes   PM practice .... minutes

The areas I worked on today:

☐ Forehead ☐ Eyes ☐ Cheeks ☐ Mouth ☐ Jaw ☐ Neck ☐ Wellness

What I am most grateful for today:

....

....

WEDNESDAY

Today's intention:

....

When I did my Face Yoga today:

AM practice .... minutes   PM practice .... minutes

The areas I worked on today:

☐ Forehead   ☐ Eyes   ☐ Cheeks   ☐ Mouth   ☐ Jaw   ☐ Neck   ☐ Wellness

What I am most grateful for today:

....

....

THURSDAY

Today's intention:

....

When I did my Face Yoga today:

AM practice .... minutes   PM practice .... minutes

The areas I worked on today:

☐ Forehead   ☐ Eyes   ☐ Cheeks   ☐ Mouth   ☐ Jaw   ☐ Neck   ☐ Wellness

What I am most grateful for today:

....

....

FRIDAY

Today's intention:

....

When I did my Face Yoga today:

AM practice .... minutes   PM practice .... minutes

The areas I worked on today:

☐ Forehead ☐ Eyes ☐ Cheeks ☐ Mouth ☐ Jaw ☐ Neck ☐ Wellness

What I am most grateful for today:

....

....

SATURDAY

Today's intention:

....

When I did my Face Yoga today:

AM practice .... minutes   PM practice .... minutes

The areas I worked on today:

☐ Forehead ☐ Eyes ☐ Cheeks ☐ Mouth ☐ Jaw ☐ Neck ☐ Wellness

What I am most grateful for today:

....

....

SUNDAY

Today's intention:

....

When I did my Face Yoga today:

AM practice .... minutes   PM practice .... minutes

The areas I worked on today:

☐ Forehead ☐ Eyes ☐ Cheeks ☐ Mouth ☐ Jaw ☐ Neck ☐ Wellness

What I am most grateful for today:

....

....

What Went Well this Week:

....

....

What Didn't Go so Well this Week:

....

....

Week 48. Calm

This week is about being calm. One of the best ways to do this is to use your mantra and focus on your root chakra. Do your Face Yoga sitting down and let yourself be rooted in the ground. Visualize a spinning wheel of red energy around the base of your spine. Really focus on your breath too this week, as this is a scientifically proven way to promote calm.

TECHNIQUE OF THE WEEK
The Eye Calming Technique

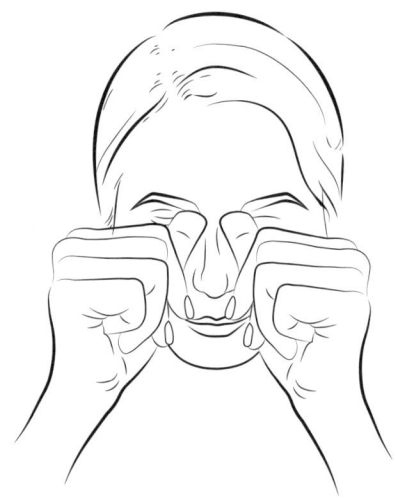

1. Place your thumbs in the inner corners of your eyes, just at the top of the nose where there is a natural indentation. Slightly tilt the head forward to put pressure on this area rather than using pressure from the thumbs. How far you tilt is up to you but don't tense or overly crease your neck. Hold for 30 seconds then release.

2. Repeat a second time if that feels right for you.

Benefits: This renowned acupressure point helps calm the mind, reduce eye strain, ease headaches and improve the *prana* or *qi* around the eye area for brighter, healthier eyes.

> **Weekly wellness hack** Reading is a calming activity to be enjoyed daily. So each day this week, read one page of a book that leaves you feeling grounded and calm.

My Positive Word for the Week:

....

The Way I Want to Feel this Week:

....

My Reason for Doing Face Yoga this Week:

....

"Stop trying to calm the storm. Calm yourself. The storm will pass."

MONDAY

Today's intention:

....

When I did my Face Yoga today:

AM practice .... minutes   PM practice .... minutes

The areas I worked on today:

☐ Forehead ☐ Eyes ☐ Cheeks ☐ Mouth ☐ Jaw ☐ Neck ☐ Wellness

What I am most grateful for today:

....

....

TUESDAY

Today's intention:

....

When I did my Face Yoga today:

AM practice .... minutes   PM practice .... minutes

The areas I worked on today:

☐ Forehead ☐ Eyes ☐ Cheeks ☐ Mouth ☐ Jaw ☐ Neck ☐ Wellness

What I am most grateful for today:

....

....

WEDNESDAY

Today's intention:

....

When I did my Face Yoga today:

AM practice .... minutes   PM practice .... minutes

The areas I worked on today:

☐ Forehead ☐ Eyes ☐ Cheeks ☐ Mouth ☐ Jaw ☐ Neck ☐ Wellness

What I am most grateful for today:

....

....

THURSDAY

Today's intention:

....

When I did my Face Yoga today:

AM practice .... minutes   PM practice .... minutes

The areas I worked on today:

☐ Forehead ☐ Eyes ☐ Cheeks ☐ Mouth ☐ Jaw ☐ Neck ☐ Wellness

What I am most grateful for today:

....

....

FRIDAY

Today's intention:

....

When I did my Face Yoga today:

AM practice .... minutes   PM practice .... minutes

The areas I worked on today:

☐ Forehead ☐ Eyes ☐ Cheeks ☐ Mouth ☐ Jaw ☐ Neck ☐ Wellness

What I am most grateful for today:

....

....

SATURDAY

Today's intention:

....

When I did my Face Yoga today:

AM practice .... minutes   PM practice .... minutes

The areas I worked on today:

☐ Forehead ☐ Eyes ☐ Cheeks ☐ Mouth ☐ Jaw ☐ Neck ☐ Wellness

What I am most grateful for today:

....

....

SUNDAY

Today's intention:

....

When I did my Face Yoga today:

AM practice .... minutes   PM practice .... minutes

The areas I worked on today:

☐ Forehead ☐ Eyes ☐ Cheeks ☐ Mouth ☐ Jaw ☐ Neck ☐ Wellness

What I am most grateful for today:

....

....

What Went Well this Week:

....

....

What Didn't Go so Well this Week:

....

....

Week 49. Blossoming

This week is about blossoming, which in essence is showing up for yourself and others as the truest, brightest and most authentic version of you. The Face Yoga technique helps the cheeks and outer nose to glow and blossom and your wellness hack is about how you can blossom into the best version of you over the coming months and years.

TECHNIQUE OF THE WEEK
The Cheek Blossoming Exercise

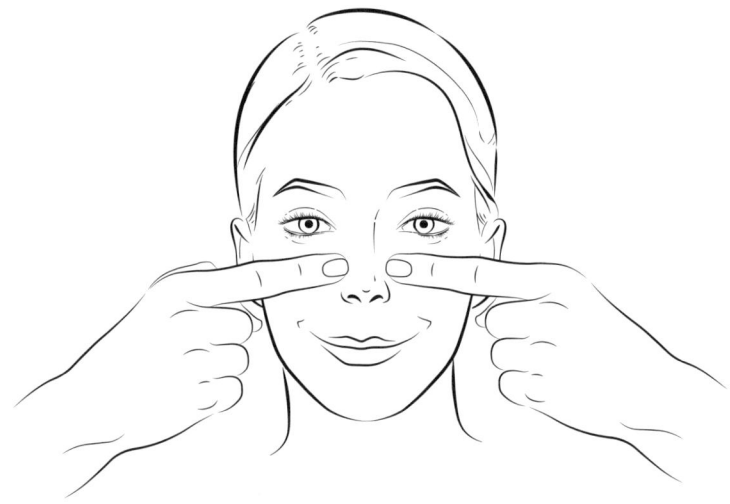

1. Place your two index fingers either side of your nose bone in a horizontal position. Flare and release your nostrils so that you engage the muscles either side of the nose and on the inner part of the cheek.

2. Continue for up to 1 minute.

Benefits: The nose is a notoriously difficult area to tone because it's mostly bone and cartilage, but you can gently tone this muscle with this lovely technique. It also helps to give a wonderful glow to the cheek area.

> **Weekly wellness hack** As you start to come to the final few weeks of your year, it's time to think about new goals for the coming year and how you can continue to blossom. To visualize this, create a vision board of pictures and words of everything you would like to do, feel, see and manifest.

My Positive Word for the Week:

....

The Way I Want to Feel this Week:

....

My Reason for Doing Face Yoga this Week:

....

"Spread your wings like a butterfly, let yourself blossom like a flower, let yourself grow like a tree."

MONDAY

Today's intention:

....

When I did my Face Yoga today:

AM practice .... minutes   PM practice .... minutes

The areas I worked on today:

☐ Forehead ☐ Eyes ☐ Cheeks ☐ Mouth ☐ Jaw ☐ Neck ☐ Wellness

What I am most grateful for today:

....

....

TUESDAY

Today's intention:

....

When I did my Face Yoga today:

AM practice .... minutes   PM practice .... minutes

The areas I worked on today:

☐ Forehead ☐ Eyes ☐ Cheeks ☐ Mouth ☐ Jaw ☐ Neck ☐ Wellness

What I am most grateful for today:

....

....

WEDNESDAY

Today's intention:

....

When I did my Face Yoga today:

AM practice .... minutes   PM practice .... minutes

The areas I worked on today:

☐ Forehead ☐ Eyes ☐ Cheeks ☐ Mouth ☐ Jaw ☐ Neck ☐ Wellness

What I am most grateful for today:

....

....

THURSDAY

Today's intention:

....

When I did my Face Yoga today:

AM practice .... minutes   PM practice .... minutes

The areas I worked on today:

☐ Forehead ☐ Eyes ☐ Cheeks ☐ Mouth ☐ Jaw ☐ Neck ☐ Wellness

What I am most grateful for today:

....

....

FRIDAY

Today's intention:

....

When I did my Face Yoga today:

AM practice .... minutes   PM practice .... minutes

The areas I worked on today:

☐ Forehead ☐ Eyes ☐ Cheeks ☐ Mouth ☐ Jaw ☐ Neck ☐ Wellness

What I am most grateful for today:

....

....

SATURDAY

Today's intention:

....

When I did my Face Yoga today:

AM practice .... minutes   PM practice .... minutes

The areas I worked on today:

☐ Forehead ☐ Eyes ☐ Cheeks ☐ Mouth ☐ Jaw ☐ Neck ☐ Wellness

What I am most grateful for today:

....

....

SUNDAY

Today's intention:

....

When I did my Face Yoga today:

AM practice .... minutes   PM practice .... minutes

The areas I worked on today:

☐ Forehead ☐ Eyes ☐ Cheeks ☐ Mouth ☐ Jaw ☐ Neck ☐ Wellness

What I am most grateful for today:

....

....

What Went Well this Week:

....

....

What Didn't Go so Well this Week:

....

....

Week 50. Unifying

Unifying means to become whole or united. In many ways, that is the whole essence of Face Yoga. This week's Face Yoga is more focused on unifying in terms of working both sides of the face together and really tuning in to your true self.

The Mouth Unifying Technique

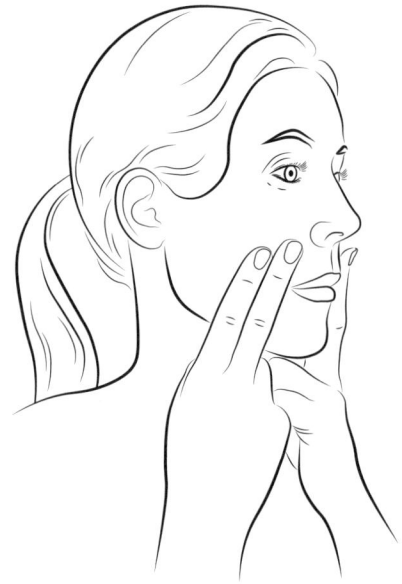

1. Press your lips together and make them into a straight line. Place your two index fingers on the line between the nostrils and the jawbone to smooth any lines created and to ensure both sides are working together. Hold your fingers and mouth in position.

2. Start to turn the head to one side, then to the other. Do this slowly, as though you are saying "no". Continue for 1 minute.

Benefits: This helps to unify both sides of the lower face, which helps with symmetry, as it encourages both sides to work together. The head turning helps to release and soothe neck tension.

Weekly wellness hack Nurture your inner child this week and do something you loved as a kid. It may be doing an activity, going to a certain place or eating a certain food. Remind yourself of the power of the innocent, carefree side of you and bring it into your adult life.

My Positive Word for the Week:

The Way I Want to Feel this Week:

My Reason for Doing Face Yoga this Week:

"*Success comes from the small steps you take each day.*"

MONDAY

Today's intention:

....

When I did my Face Yoga today:

AM practice .... minutes   PM practice .... minutes

The areas I worked on today:

☐ Forehead ☐ Eyes ☐ Cheeks ☐ Mouth ☐ Jaw ☐ Neck ☐ Wellness

What I am most grateful for today:

....

....

TUESDAY

Today's intention:

....

When I did my Face Yoga today:

AM practice .... minutes   PM practice .... minutes

The areas I worked on today:

☐ Forehead ☐ Eyes ☐ Cheeks ☐ Mouth ☐ Jaw ☐ Neck ☐ Wellness

What I am most grateful for today:

....

....

WEDNESDAY

Today's intention:

....

When I did my Face Yoga today:

AM practice .... minutes   PM practice .... minutes

The areas I worked on today:

☐ Forehead ☐ Eyes ☐ Cheeks ☐ Mouth ☐ Jaw ☐ Neck ☐ Wellness

What I am most grateful for today:

....

....

THURSDAY

Today's intention:

....

When I did my Face Yoga today:

AM practice .... minutes   PM practice .... minutes

The areas I worked on today:

☐ Forehead ☐ Eyes ☐ Cheeks ☐ Mouth ☐ Jaw ☐ Neck ☐ Wellness

What I am most grateful for today:

....

....

FRIDAY

Today's intention:

....

When I did my Face Yoga today:

AM practice .... minutes   PM practice .... minutes

The areas I worked on today:

☐ Forehead ☐ Eyes ☐ Cheeks ☐ Mouth ☐ Jaw ☐ Neck ☐ Wellness

What I am most grateful for today:

....

....

SATURDAY

Today's intention:

....

When I did my Face Yoga today:

AM practice .... minutes   PM practice .... minutes

The areas I worked on today:

☐ Forehead ☐ Eyes ☐ Cheeks ☐ Mouth ☐ Jaw ☐ Neck ☐ Wellness

What I am most grateful for today:

....

....

SUNDAY

Today's intention:

....

When I did my Face Yoga today:

AM practice .... minutes   PM practice .... minutes

The areas I worked on today:

☐ Forehead ☐ Eyes ☐ Cheeks ☐ Mouth ☐ Jaw ☐ Neck ☐ Wellness

What I am most grateful for today:

....

....

What Went Well this Week:

....

....

What Didn't Go so Well this Week:

....

....

Week 51. Balance

I f there is one word I would like you to take with you as you complete your journey this year, it's balance. As you go forward, either by doing this journal again or using another means, always look for balance in every area of your life. This will serve you well.

TECHNIQUE OF THE WEEK
The Jaw Balancing Technique

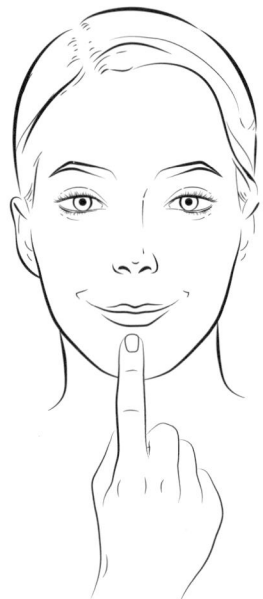

1. Using gentle yet firm pressure, press the indent of your chin with the index finger of one hand and massage in a circular motion in one direction for 30 seconds.

2. Massage in the other direction for 30 seconds.

Benefits: In facial reflexology (which links each acupressure point on the face with an organ or system in the body) this point is renowned to help the bowels, relieve constipation and reduce dull facial skin.

Weekly wellness hack Give yourself some grace this week. Over the last year you have done so many positive wellness and Face Yoga techniques, but also no doubt, you have eaten, felt or done things which aren't always great for your face, body and mind. This week simply tell yourself "I am enough" and remind yourself life is about balance and its okay to not be perfect.

My Positive Word for the Week:

....

The Way I Want to Feel this Week:

....

My Reason for Doing Face Yoga this Week:

....

"You reached here by taking one step at a time and finding balance. You will reach where you need to be next in the same way."

MONDAY

Today's intention:

....

When I did my Face Yoga today:

AM practice .... minutes   PM practice .... minutes

The areas I worked on today:

☐ Forehead ☐ Eyes ☐ Cheeks ☐ Mouth ☐ Jaw ☐ Neck ☐ Wellness

What I am most grateful for today:

....

....

TUESDAY

Today's intention:

....

When I did my Face Yoga today:

AM practice .... minutes   PM practice .... minutes

The areas I worked on today:

☐ Forehead ☐ Eyes ☐ Cheeks ☐ Mouth ☐ Jaw ☐ Neck ☐ Wellness

What I am most grateful for today:

....

....

WEDNESDAY

Today's intention:

....

When I did my Face Yoga today:

AM practice .... minutes   PM practice .... minutes

The areas I worked on today:

☐ Forehead ☐ Eyes ☐ Cheeks ☐ Mouth ☐ Jaw ☐ Neck ☐ Wellness

What I am most grateful for today:

....

....

THURSDAY

Today's intention:

....

When I did my Face Yoga today:

AM practice .... minutes   PM practice .... minutes

The areas I worked on today:

☐ Forehead ☐ Eyes ☐ Cheeks ☐ Mouth ☐ Jaw ☐ Neck ☐ Wellness

What I am most grateful for today:

....

....

FRIDAY

Today's intention:

....

When I did my Face Yoga today:

AM practice .... minutes   PM practice .... minutes

The areas I worked on today:

☐ Forehead ☐ Eyes ☐ Cheeks ☐ Mouth ☐ Jaw ☐ Neck ☐ Wellness

What I am most grateful for today:

....

....

SATURDAY

Today's intention:

....

When I did my Face Yoga today:

AM practice .... minutes   PM practice .... minutes

The areas I worked on today:

☐ Forehead ☐ Eyes ☐ Cheeks ☐ Mouth ☐ Jaw ☐ Neck ☐ Wellness

What I am most grateful for today:

....

....

SUNDAY

Today's intention:

....

When I did my Face Yoga today:

AM practice .... minutes   PM practice .... minutes

The areas I worked on today:

☐ Forehead ☐ Eyes ☐ Cheeks ☐ Mouth ☐ Jaw ☐ Neck ☐ Wellness

What I am most grateful for today:

....

....

What Went Well this Week:

....

....

What Didn't Go so Well this Week:

....

....

Week 52. Celebration

You deserve to celebrate! At the end of this last week you will have dedicated 12 months, 52 weeks, to Face Yoga, to wellness and to yourself. To complete your journal, this week's technique is a wonderful pose that opens the throat chakra as well as helps you feel jubilant. You can focus on congratulating yourself but also be reflective of the journey you have been on.

TECHNIQUE OF THE WEEK
The Neck Celebrating Technique

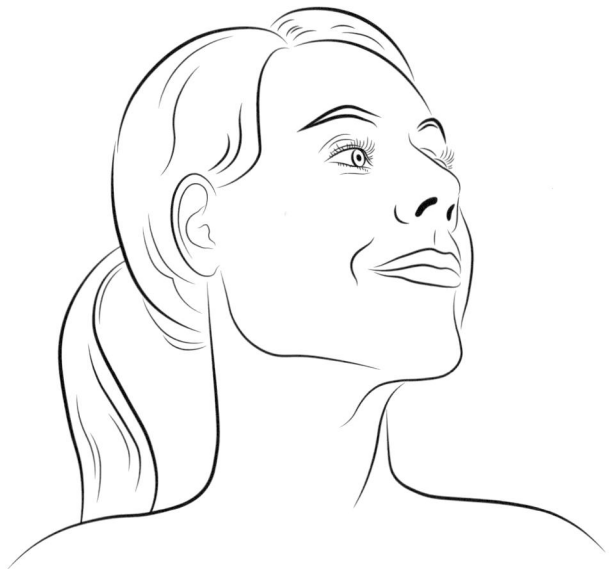

1. Open your arms out wide like big wings and gently tilt your head back so that your chin is pointing upward slightly – only as far as is comfortable for you.

2. Move your head from side to side with a slight smile on your face (keeping the rest of your face in neutral) and feel a sense of pride and celebration.

Benefits: This helps to relieve tight shoulders, chest and neck and therefore soothes away stress and tension from the face.

> **Weekly wellness hack** For the next seven days treat yourself daily. This can be with a selection of the wellness hacks you have done this year or with other ways. The goal is to celebrate in a healthy way and, most of all, to feel good!

My Positive Word for the Week:

....

The Way I Want to Feel this Week:

....

My Reason for Doing Face Yoga this Week:

....

"Take a moment to notice how far you have come."

MONDAY

Today's intention:

....

When I did my Face Yoga today:

AM practice .... minutes   PM practice .... minutes

The areas I worked on today:

☐ Forehead ☐ Eyes ☐ Cheeks ☐ Mouth ☐ Jaw ☐ Neck ☐ Wellness

What I am most grateful for today:

....

....

TUESDAY

Today's intention:

....

When I did my Face Yoga today:

AM practice .... minutes   PM practice .... minutes

The areas I worked on today:

☐ Forehead ☐ Eyes ☐ Cheeks ☐ Mouth ☐ Jaw ☐ Neck ☐ Wellness

What I am most grateful for today:

....

....

WEDNESDAY

Today's intention:

....

When I did my Face Yoga today:

AM practice .... minutes   PM practice .... minutes

The areas I worked on today:

☐ Forehead ☐ Eyes ☐ Cheeks ☐ Mouth ☐ Jaw ☐ Neck ☐ Wellness

What I am most grateful for today:

....

....

THURSDAY

Today's intention:

....

When I did my Face Yoga today:

AM practice .... minutes   PM practice .... minutes

The areas I worked on today:

☐ Forehead ☐ Eyes ☐ Cheeks ☐ Mouth ☐ Jaw ☐ Neck ☐ Wellness

What I am most grateful for today:

....

....

FRIDAY

Today's intention:

....

When I did my Face Yoga today:

AM practice .... minutes   PM practice .... minutes

The areas I worked on today:

☐ Forehead ☐ Eyes ☐ Cheeks ☐ Mouth ☐ Jaw ☐ Neck ☐ Wellness

What I am most grateful for today:

....

....

SATURDAY

Today's intention:

....

When I did my Face Yoga today:

AM practice .... minutes   PM practice .... minutes

The areas I worked on today:

☐ Forehead ☐ Eyes ☐ Cheeks ☐ Mouth ☐ Jaw ☐ Neck ☐ Wellness

What I am most grateful for today:

....

....

SUNDAY

Today's intention:

....

When I did my Face Yoga today:

AM practice .... minutes   PM practice .... minutes

The areas I worked on today:

☐ Forehead   ☐ Eyes   ☐ Cheeks   ☐ Mouth   ☐ Jaw   ☐ Neck   ☐ Wellness

What I am most grateful for today:

....

....

What Went Well this Week:

....

....

What Didn't Go so Well this Week:

....

....

The End of the Year

You have done it! A huge well done for finishing your journal. You should be so proud. A full year of daily Face Yoga and wellness is fantastic. I would highly recommend taking a little glance through the journal at what you have written over each of the weeks and seasons. Use this firstly as a reminder of how far you have come and the progress you have made. Secondly, look at where you wrote down what didn't go well in a week or found it hard to complete a week and use those as a reminder that you are human and progress is also better than perfection.

Now you may be thinking, what next? Here are a few suggestions for how to continue:

- Do another journal. Quite simply, start with a fresh unused journal and continue for another year. There will be so many benefits to doing this (and you will find different benefits year on year). I highly recommend making it a habit for life.
- Use this same journal to prompt you for your Face Yoga each week. This won't be quite as effective as you won't have clear space to record progress and journal your thoughts and feelings, but it will still mean you are doing daily Face Yoga, which is great.
- Use my first book, *Danielle Collins' Face Yoga* (also available as a 10-day course, an audio book and digital version) and use this to enjoy Face Yoga.
- Use any of my other courses, apps or DVDs.

For information on all the above, head to faceyogaexpert.com.

And finally, a few words to take you on your way. When you doubt yourself, please know this: you are stronger, braver and more beautiful than you ever know. Also I want to say thank you. Thank you for coming on this journey with me. I wrote this with love and a desire deep in my soul to help you feel healthier and happier each day.

Oh, and one last piece of advice: don't forget to keep wearing your SPF daily, drink lots of water, get eight hours sleep and, most of all, feel gratitude for your face, body, mind and life.

From my heart and soul to yours,

Danielle